The WHAT *to* EAT
if YOU HAVE
DIABETES
COOKBOOK

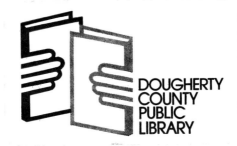

DOUGHERTY
COUNTY
PUBLIC
LIBRARY

The WHAT *to* EAT *if* YOU HAVE DIABETES COOKBOOK

*Simple, Balanced Recipes
and Meal Plans*

**MAUREEN KEANE, M.S., AND
DANIELLA CHACE, M.S.**

CB
CONTEMPORARY BOOKS

Library of Congress Cataloging-in-Publication Data

Keane, Maureen, 1950–.
    The what to eat if you have diabetes cookbook : simple, balanced
recipes and meal plans / Maureen Keane and Daniella Chace.
      p.   cm.
    Includes index.
    ISBN 0-8092-2817-3
    1. Diabetes—Diet therapy—Recipes.   I. Chace, Daniella.
II. Title.
RC662.K43   1999
641.5′6314—dc21   98-44793
                                         CIP

Published by Contemporary Books
A division of NTC/Contemporary Publishing Group, Inc.
4255 West Touhy Avenue, Lincolnwood (Chicago), Illinois 60646-1975 U.S.A.
Copyright © 1999 by Daniella Chace and Maureen Keane
All rights reserved. No part of this book may be reproduced, stored in a retrieval
system, or transmitted in any form or by any means, electronic, mechanical,
photocopying, recording, or otherwise, without the prior permission of
NTC/Contemporary Publishing Group, Inc.
Printed in the United States of America
International Standard Book Number: 0-8092-2817-3

99 00 01 02 03 04 QP 19 18 17 16 15 14 13 12 11 10 9 8 7 6 5 4 3 2 1

Contents

Acknowledgments

The authors give their deepest appreciation to Linda Landkamer for her recipe development and testing; LaMar Harrington for the use of her beautiful beachside test kitchen in Port Townsend; Michelle LaRock for her nutrition analysis expertise; our recipe-testing crew: Gary Boyer, Michael Levine, Darci Chace, Lynn Wilson, and Linda Landkamer; Dr. Bruce Milliman; our copyeditor: Gerilee Hundt; and our project editor: Heidi Bresnahan.

We also wish to thank Spectrum Naturals for providing organic oils for our test kitchen and the Zyliss Kitchen Tools company for providing the latest version of their fabulous Suzi garlic press.

Introduction

This cookbook is intended to be used as a companion volume to *What to Eat if You Have Diabetes* (NTC/Contemporary, 1999). *What to Eat if You Have Diabetes* explains the "why" to the diet, and it includes the blank forms needed for recording your dietary information. The individualized program was developed to simplify the task of recording blood-sugar readings, insulin, medication, and supplement intake information. The individualized program defined in *What to Eat if You Have Diabetes* provides one simple form for recording all this as well as food intake.

Our dietary recommendations are based on the healthful benefits of natural whole foods. These foods include fish, natural herbal sweeteners, and legumes (beans, peas, and lentils). Legumes have powerful blood-sugar-regulating properties and are naturally high in fiber, protein, and complex carbohydrates. Nature has conveniently packaged these hearty foods with approximately 50 percent carbohydrate and 25 percent protein. The remaining 25 percent of the daily calories are in the form of healthful fat including essential fatty acids. This 50/25/25 macronutrient ratio is advised for blood-sugar regulation.

The foods that make up the recipes in this book should be as unprocessed and as unadulterated as possible. This means that these foods contain no food additives or preservatives and are not genetically altered. Always choose organic foods, as they are the only foods on our grocery store shelves that are guaranteed to be grown without pesticides, herbicides, genetic alteration, or irradiation.

These recipes are not all vegetarian, but there are very few animal products used. Animal products contain no fiber, are often tainted with hormones such as bovine growth hormone, and generally contain unhealthy fats.

Foods known to help stabilize blood sugar are used to create recipes that fit into the 50/25/25 plan. This plan allows you to have three meals (breakfast, lunch, and dinner) and one snack a day. As with any healthful diet plan, keep your dessert intake to a minimum. When you want to indulge your sweet tooth, you will find many enticing recipes in Chapter 6.

The dietary guidelines used to create these recipes are as follows.

- Fifty percent of total daily calories come from such carbohydrate foods as beans, peas, and lentils, vegetables, sea vegetables, whole grains, and fruits.
- Twenty-five percent of total daily calories come from protein sources such as beans, peas, and lentils, nuts and seeds, fish and shellfish, and soy foods (tofu, tempeh, soy flour, and soy milk).
- Twenty-five percent of total daily calories come from fats in the form of fish, nuts, seeds, and oils such as flaxseed oil, extra-virgin olive oil, and fish oil.
- Dairy foods are used minimally and only as condiments. Minimize dairy foods such as milk, butter, and cream. Include only nonfat yogurt, cheese, and eggs to an intake of 5 percent or less of total daily calories (i.e., 75 calories in a 1,500 calorie diet).
- Avoid refined foods such as white sugar and refined breads, pastas, and baked goods made with white flour.
- Eliminate unhealthful foods such as red meat, synthetic sweeteners, synthetic fats, lard, and hydrogenated oils.
- Include spices and herbs such as holy basil, stevia, and licorice root and phytochemically rich foods such as garlic, onions, and bitter melon.
- Eat only organic foods whenever possible.

- Drink and cook with purified water.

We have constructed the following meals (using the recipes in this book) to meet the caloric requirements for a 1,500-calorie diet. Each meal contains approximately 450 calories and each snack contains approximately 150 calories. See Macronutrient chart on page xviii for directions as to modifying this menu plan to fit other caloric requirements (1,200; 1,750; 2,000; and so on).

The following combinations equal 450 calories and are complete meals:

Breakfast
- Tofu Waffles and 6 servings of Blueberry Sauce
- Tofu Waffles, 3 servings of Maple Syrup, and 2 tablespoons walnuts
- Tofu Scramble, Strawberry Squares, and a Licorice Smoothie
- Blueberry Pancake and Waffle Mix, 6 servings of Blueberry Sauce, and a Raspberry Vanilla Smoothie
- Banana Smoothie and Tofu Scramble
- Muesli with fruit and soy milk

Lunch / Dinner
- Chicken and Pesto Dinner
- Spicy Basil Chicken
- Lentil and Arame Stew
- Black-Eyed Peas with Sun-Dried Tomatoes
- Fish and Eggplant Curry, 2 cups of Licorice Root Tea, and Banana-Blueberry Cream Pie
- Blackened Catfish; Hijiki, Tofu, and Ginger Salad; and 1 Nori Roll
- Blackened Catfish, 2 servings of Tartar Sauce, 2 servings of Baked Herb Fries, and 3 servings of Tofu Ketchup
- Hijiki Salad, a large bowl of Miso and Tofu Soup (2 servings), and Hijiki and Shiitake Mushrooms

- Curried Tuna Salad, Colesaw, and Licorice Root Tea
- Edamame and Holy Basil Salad, Herbed Fish with Spicy Salsa, 2 servings of Tartar Sauce, and Fenugreek Tea
- Kombu-Squash Soup, Nori Rolls, Edamame, Cabbage Riata, and Green Tea
- Eggless Caesar Salad with Chicken, Roasted Eggplant and Mozzarella Sandwich, and 1 Power Cookie
- Greek Salad and Licorice Smoothie
- Asian Salad, Marinated Tofu, Toasted Nori Squares, and Green Tea
- Creamy Tomato Pasta and 3 servings of Tofu Meatballs
- White Bean Salad, Spicy Corn Bread, and Chocolate Mousse
- Chinese Cabbage and Dulse Soup, Snow Peas with Wakame Dressing, Strawberry Squares, and 2 servings of Whipped Cream
- Spiced Cream of Pumpkin Soup and Coleslaw
- Lentil Stew and Baked Pears
- Spicy Quinoa Pilaf with Fish, Vanilla Pudding
- White Beans and Green Herb Salad, Asian Kombu Potato Sauté, and Creamy Chinese Soup
- Baked Potatoes with Onion Sauce, Jicama and Holy Basil Salad, and Vegetable Curry
- Wilted Asian Hijiki Salad, Baked Root Vegetables, 2 servings Gazpacho, and 1 Power Cookie
- Enchiladas and Red Sauce and 1 cup raw spinach leaves with 1 serving Kumquat Dressing
- Marinated Tuna, Arame with Onions, Spicy Japanese Broth, and Chocolate Mousse
- Baked Beans, Spicy Corn Bread, and Green Tea
- Beans, Greens, and Grains and Baked Pears
- Beans, Greens, and Grains; Herbed Soup; Licorice Root Tea; and Chocolate Mousse
- Beans, Greens, and Grains; Arame-Stuffed Mushrooms; and Chocolate Banana Milk Shake

- Asian Kombu Potato Sauté, Asian Arame dressing over 1 cup raw spinach, and Fruit Gel

The following snacks contain the ideal 150 calories.

- Popcorn with nutritional yeast
- Soy Yogurt and Apricots
- Vanilla Licorice Shake
- Edamame (4 ounces)

Many of the recipes are interchangeable to make daily meal planning easier. Most of the ingredients are easily found at most grocery stores. There are a few ingredients we found to be of such profound benefit that, even though they will have to be purchased at a health-food store or co-op or ordered through the mail, we feel you'll be glad that you searched them out. For those products we recommend, we have listed purchasing sources in the Resources section at the end of the book. Each ingredient has been thoroughly reviewed and analyzed with nutrition analysis software to be sure that these recipes will provide the greatest blood-sugar-regulating benefit possible.

With each delicious bite, you can rest assured that you are enhancing your health by reducing your chances of developing heart disease, strengthening your immune system, and providing the right fuel for lean weight maintenance, all while caring for your diabetes.

Enjoy!
Daniella Chace
Maureen Keane

Macronutrient Ratios
for Individual Caloric Allowances

Based on 3 equal meals + 1 snack
(50% carbohydrates, 25% protein, 25% fat)

Meals

DAILY CALORIC ALLOWANCE	CALORIES PER MEAL	CARBOHYDRATES		PROTEIN		FAT	
		Calories	Grams	Calories	Grams	Calories	Grams
1,200	360	180	45	90	22	90	10
1,500	450	225	56	112	28	112	12
1,750	525	262	65	131	32	131	14.5
2,000	600	300	75	150	37	150	16
2,250	675	337	84	168	42	168	18.5
2,500	750	375	93	187	46	187	20

Snacks

DAILY CALORIC ALLOWANCE	CALORIES PER SNACK	CARBOHYDRATES		PROTEIN		FAT	
		Calories	Grams	Calories	Grams	Calories	Grams
1,200	120	67	16	33	8	33	3.5
1,500	150	73	19	37	9	37	4
1,750	175	87	21	43	10	43	4.5
2,000	200	100	25	50	12	50	5.5
2,250	225	112	28	56	14	56	6
2,500	250	125	31	62	15	62	6.5

The WHAT *to* EAT *if* YOU HAVE DIABETES COOKBOOK

I

Breakfast

Tofu Scramble

....

1 tablespoon extra-virgin olive oil
½ sweet onion, chopped
½ pound firm tofu
¼ teaspoon turmeric
¼ cup chopped fresh basil leaves
¼ cup grated soy Parmesan cheese

1. Heat the olive oil in a medium skillet.
2. Add the onion and sauté until the onion becomes translucent.
3. Crumble the tofu into the skillet and sprinkle the turmeric over the top. Mix well. The turmeric gives the tofu a yellow egglike color. Cook the tofu until it begins to brown.
4. Add the basil leaves and Parmesan cheese. Cover and heat for another 5 minutes.
5. Serve hot.

⌁ Makes 2 servings

NUTRITIONAL INFORMATION PER SERVING

Calories 140	Carbohydrate 8g
Fat 7g	Fiber 2g
Cholesterol 0mg	Protein 12g

Tofu Waffles

1 cup whole-grain waffle mix
¼ to ½ cup soy milk
1 large egg
½ cup firm tofu
1 teaspoon vanilla extract
1 tablespoon ground flaxseed
2 tablespoons chopped walnuts

1. Spray a waffle iron with canola oil, then heat up the waffle iron.
2. Place all ingredients in a blender and blend until smooth.
3. Let the batter sit for 5 minutes after blending to allow the flaxseed to thicken the batter.
4. Pour the batter into the waffle iron and cook until steam stops rising.
5. Serve hot with Maple Syrup, Blueberry Sauce, Fruit Gel, or Cherry Breakfast Spread (see Index for recipes).

Makes 4 servings

NUTRITIONAL INFORMATION PER SERVING

Calories 360

Carbohydrate 54g

Fat 11g

Fiber 1g

Cholesterol 55mg

Protein 12g

Blueberry Pancake and Waffle Mix

....

This batter works well for pancakes or waffles and can be made in advance and stored until you need it. Wet batter will store up to three days in a well-sealed container in the refrigerator. You may also mix the dry ingredients and store in plastic bags or other well-sealed containers in the freezer for several months. When you are ready to make the batter, simply add the oil, water, and blueberries.

2 cups whole wheat or barley flour
½ cup nonfat soy milk powder
4 teaspoons baking powder
1 teaspoon salt
¼ cup canola oil
¼ cup water
½ cup fresh or frozen blueberries

1. Combine the flour, soy milk powder, baking powder, and salt in a large bowl and mix well.
2. Slowly add the oil and water, mixing constantly until it is completely absorbed.
3. Gently fold in blueberries
4. Follow directions below for making pancakes or waffles.

5. Serve hot with Maple Syrup, Blueberry Sauce, Fruit Gel, or Cherry Breakfast Spread (see Index).

∼ Makes 4 servings

Directions for Pancake

1. Using a measuring cup, pour batter onto a hot, oiled griddle, spacing the pancakes at equal intervals.
2. Cook pancakes on both sides until golden brown.

Directions for Waffles

1. Preheat waffle iron and brush (or spray) lightly with oil if necessary.
2. Pour in just enough batter to fill iron.
3. Close and cook until steaming stops and waffles are crisp.

NUTRITIONAL INFORMATION PER SERVING

Calories 370	Carbohydrate 48g
Fat 15g	Fiber 8g
Cholesterol omg	Protein 9g

Muesli

....

½ pound rolled oats
½ pound oat bran
¼ pound lecithin granules
¼ pound flaxseed, ground in a coffee grinder
⅛ pound raw pumpkin seeds
¼ pound filberts (hazelnuts)
⅛ pound pecans
6 ounces wheat germ
½ cup tap water (room temperature)
6 cups light soy milk (vanilla flavor)
6 cups fresh strawberries

1. Mix together the oats, oat bran, lecithin, flaxseed, pumpkin seeds, nuts, and wheat germ in a large bowl or paper bag.
2. Soak ½ cup muesli in water for at least ½ hour before serving. Add ½ cup soy milk and ½ cup berries to each serving.
3. Store unused muesli in plastic bags or containers in the freezer; it will keep for about 1 month.

Makes 12 servings

NUTRITIONAL INFORMATION PER SERVING

Calories 450	Carbohydrate 38g
Fat 27g	Fiber 7g
Cholesterol 5mg	Protein 13g

Cherry Breakfast Spread

3 tablespoons agar flakes
4 cups apple juice
2½ cups pureed fresh ripe cherries
1 teaspoon fresh lemon juice

1. Pour the agar, apple juice, and cherries into a saucepan and heat over medium heat.
2. Simmer for 5 minutes, then stir in the lemon juice.
3. Pour into a mold or a glass container with a lid and allow the gel to set, about 10 minutes. Spread on toast, waffles, or pancakes.

Makes 18 servings

NUTRITIONAL INFORMATION PER SERVING

Calories 50	Carbohydrate 12g
Fat 0g	Fiber 1g
Cholesterol 0mg	Protein 0g

2

Lunch

Bean Dip

....

2 cups prepared refried beans (nonfat beans)
1 tablespoon flaxseed oil
1 cup chunky salsa
¼ cup chopped cilantro
1 ripe avocado, chopped

1. Combine all ingredients in a medium bowl and mix well.
2. Serve with baked corn chips or raw vegetables for dipping.

~ *Makes 4 servings*

Note: Only purchase beans that have no added oil or lard. Look for the labels that state "low-fat," "nonfat," or "vegetarian."

NUTRITIONAL INFORMATION PER SERVING

Calories 240	Carbohydrate 23g
Fat 11g	Fiber 10g
Cholesterol 10mg	Protein 12g

Creamy Hummus

....

1 16-ounce can garbanzo beans
Juice of 2 lemons
1 teaspoon sea salt
½ cup water
3 tablespoons flaxseed oil
4 cloves garlic
½ cup tahini
1 teaspoon chopped fresh mint

1. In a blender or food processor, puree together the garbanzo beans, lemon juice, salt, water, oil, garlic, and tahini until creamy.
2. Stir in the mint and serve with toasted pita wedges, raw vegetables, or crackers. This spread is also delicious on sandwiches.

∼ Makes 10 servings

NUTRITIONAL INFORMATION PER SERVING

Calories 110	Carbohydrate 9g
Fat 6g	Fiber 2g
Cholesterol 0mg	Protein 3g

Hijiki Salad

1 teaspoon sesame oil *or* ½ cup water
1 cup hijiki, reconstituted in water, drained, and chopped
2 tablespoons rice vinegar
1 teaspoon fresh lemon juice
1 carrot, grated
5 mushrooms, chopped
¼ yellow onion, chopped

1. Heat the oil or water in a skillet until very hot.
2. Sauté the hijiki in the oil or water for 20 to 30 minutes. Allow to cool.
3. Mix all ingredients together and serve over chopped greens.

~ *Makes 4 servings*

Hijiki

Hijiki is a popular Asian sea vegetable with a nutlike flavor and crisp texture. The fresh clean plants are dried and sold in bulk and in packages through Asian markets and health-food stores. Hijiki is delicious and nutritionally rich in protein, B vitamins, calcium, phosphorus, iron, and trace elements. The dried hijiki should be hydrated first in fresh water and then drained before cooking.

NUTRITIONAL INFORMATION PER SERVING

Calories 30	Carbohydrate 6g
Fat 0g	Fiber 4g
Cholesterol 0mg	Protein 0g

Hijiki, Tofu, and Ginger Salad

....

2 teaspoons sesame seeds

1 tablespoon toasted sesame oil

1½ cups dried hijiki, reconstituted in water, drained, and rinsed

1 cup cubed firm tofu

3 carrots, shredded

1 tablespoon grated fresh gingerroot

1½ teaspoons tamari or soy sauce

1 tablespoon mirin

1. Roast the sesame seeds in a dry skillet over medium heat just until they begin to brown. Remove from heat and set aside.
2. Heat the oil in a large saucepan. Add the hijiki and sauté over medium heat for 5 minutes. Add the tofu, carrots, and ginger to the pan and cook for another 5 minutes. Remove the pan from heat. Add the tamari, mirin, and sesame seeds and toss.
3. Serve hot or cold.

~ *Makes 4 servings*

NUTRITIONAL INFORMATION PER SERVING

Calories 160

Fat 10g

Cholesterol 0mg

Carbohydrate 8g

Fiber 6g

Protein 10g

Wilted Asian Hijiki Salad

1 tablespoon sesame oil
1 1-inch piece fresh gingerroot, peeled and minced
2 cloves garlic, minced
½ cup hijiki, reconstituted in 2 cups water, drained
1 tablespoon tamari or soy sauce

1. Heat the sesame oil in a skillet. Add the ginger and garlic and cook over low heat for 2 minutes.
2. Add the drained hijiki and cook for 5 minutes more.
3. Add the tamari and cook for 3 more minutes.
4. Serve each person 2 tablespoons as a warm side salad or as a topping for rice.

Makes 6 servings

NUTRITIONAL INFORMATION PER SERVING

Calories 30	Carbohydrate 2g
Fat 2.5g	Fiber 1g
Cholesterol 0mg	Protein 0g

Asian Salad

....

1 pound organic green soybeans, steamed and shelled
1 pound firm tofu, diced
2 fresh ripe tomatoes, chopped
½ cup mung bean sprouts
2 scallions, sliced
1 cup chopped Italian parsley
2 tablespoons sesame seeds
1 tablespoon minced yellow onion
Juice of ½ lemon
1 tablespoon balsamic vinegar
1 teaspoon sesame oil
1 teaspoon tamari or soy sauce

1. Place the soybeans in a steamer or saucepan and steam until soft, 5 to 8 minutes.
2. Place the tofu, tomatoes, sprouts, scallions, parsley, sesame seeds, and onion in a large bowl and toss together. Squeeze the lemon juice over the salad and sprinkle with the vinegar, sesame oil, and tamari. Toss well.
3. Add the steamed soybeans and toss again.
4. Serve immediately.

Makes 4 servings

NUTRITIONAL INFORMATION PER SERVING

Calories 350

Carbohydrate 13g

Fat 20g

Fiber 5g

Cholesterol 0mg

Protein 29g

Jicama and Holy Basil Salad

1 jicama, grated
1 carrot, grated
½ cup holy basil leaves
¼ jalapeño pepper, grated
¼ cup chopped fresh mint leaves
1 tablespoon fresh lime juice

1. Toss all ingredients together in a large bowl.
2. Serve immediately.

∼ Makes 4 servings

Holy Basil

Holy Basil is known as tulsi *in India and* bai gaprao *in Thailand. Many Hindus grow this revered holy plant in their homes. It is used extensively in Thai cooking for its hot peppery taste.*

NUTRITIONAL INFORMATION PER SERVING

Calories 35	Carbohydrate 7g
Fat 0g	Fiber 4g
Cholesterol 0mg	Protein 1g

Edamame and Holy Basil Salad

1 pound organic green soybeans, steamed and shelled
1 bunch spinach, chard, or mixed wild greens
½ cup chopped holy basil leaves
1 red bell pepper, seeded and chopped
Dash of sea salt
½ teaspoon fresh lemon juice
3 tablespoons crumbled feta cheese

1. Steam the soybeans, then chill them.
2. Wash the greens, dry them in a salad spinner or on a paper towel, and chop.
3. Toss together all ingredients.
4. Serve chilled.

◠ Makes 4 servings

Note: Holy basil has been found to help maintain blood sugar levels in non-insulin-dependent diabetes.

NUTRITIONAL INFORMATION PER SERVING

Calories 220	Carbohydrate 8g
Fat 12g	Fiber 5g
Cholesterol 5mg	Protein 20g

Cabbage Riata

1 cup plain nonfat yogurt
½ teaspoon sea salt
1 teaspoon ground cumin
½ pound cabbage, shredded
¼ teaspoon cayenne (optional)

1. Place all ingredients together in a large bowl and toss until well mixed.
2. Serve immediately or chill in the refrigerator.

Makes 4 servings

NUTRITIONAL INFORMATION PER SERVING

Calories 50

Fat 0g

Cholesterol 0mg

Carbohydrate 8g

Fiber 1g

Protein 4g

Greek Salad

2 fresh ripe tomatoes, chopped
1 cucumber, peeled and chopped
2 tablespoons capers
2 Greek olives, chopped
½ teaspoon crushed dried oregano
1 tablespoon extra-virgin olive oil
½ cup crumbled herbed tofu
1 tablespoon balsamic vinegar
Juice of ½ lemon

1. Toss all ingredients together in a large bowl.
2. Serve immediately.

Makes 2 servings

NUTRITIONAL INFORMATION PER SERVING

Calories 220	Carbohydrate 13g
Fat 13g	Fiber 4g
Cholesterol 0mg	Protein 12g

White Bean Salad

1 14-ounce can white beans, drained
1 cup chopped fresh Italian parsley
2 fresh ripe tomatoes, chopped
½ red onion, minced
Juice of ½ lemon
2 tablespoons balsamic vinegar
¼ teaspoon freshly ground sea salt
1 tablespoon extra-virgin olive oil

1. Place all ingredients in a large bowl and mix together thoroughly.
2. Serve chilled.

Makes 4 servings

NUTRITIONAL INFORMATION PER SERVING

Calories 120	Carbohydrate 17g
Fat 4g	Fiber 6g
Cholesterol 0mg	Protein 5g

Curried Tuna Salad

....

1 6-ounce can tuna packed in water, drained

2 cloves garlic, minced

1 tablespoon fresh lemon juice

1 tablespoon curry powder

1 tablespoon mayonnaise

Pinch of black pepper

Pinch of sea salt

2 whole wheat pitas

1. Place all ingredients in a medium bowl and mix together thoroughly.
2. Stuff the pitas with the filling.
3. Serve with sliced cabbage, spinach, green peppers, and tomatoes, if desired.

Makes 2 servings

NUTRITIONAL INFORMATION PER SERVING

Calories 325	Carbohydrate 38g
Fat 8g	Fiber 5g
Cholesterol 30mg	Protein 28g

Eggless Caesar Salad with Chicken

2 boneless, skinless chicken breasts
3 tablespoons flaxseed oil
¼ cup fresh lemon juice
3 cloves garlic, minced or crushed
¼ teaspoon sea salt
1 head romaine, chopped
¼ cup freshly grated Parmesan cheese

1. Place the chicken breasts in a nonstick pan and heat over medium heat. Cover and cook until the chicken is no longer pink and is completely cooked. Set aside.
2. In large bowl, combine the flaxseed oil, lemon juice, garlic, and salt. Mix well.
3. Shred the chicken into bite-size pieces and add, along with the lettuce, to the bowl. Toss with the dressing and grated Parmesan.

Makes 4 servings

NUTRITIONAL INFORMATION PER SERVING

Calories 230	Carbohydrate 1g
Fat 11g	Fiber 1g
Cholesterol 75mg	Protein 29g

Creamy Tomato Soup

....

1 pound silken or smooth tofu, crumbled
3 cups spicy tomato juice
2 cloves garlic, minced
Freshly ground black pepper

1. Place the tofu, tomato juice, and garlic in a blender and process until smooth and creamy.
2. Pour into a saucepan and simmer over low heat just until hot.
3. Serve topped with pepper.

Makes 6 servings

NUTRITIONAL INFORMATION PER SERVING

Calories 150	Carbohydrate 9g
Fat 7g	Fiber 2g
Cholesterol 0mg	Protein 13g

Miso and Tofu Soup

1 tablespoon extra-virgin olive oil

1 pound firm organic tofu, diced

4 cups water

4 tablespoons miso paste

2 scallions, sliced

1. Heat the olive oil in a skillet.
2. Add the tofu and sauté until browned.
3. Heat the water in a saucepan over low heat.
4. Dissolve the miso paste into the water, then add the scallions and sautéed tofu. Warm gently for 3 to 5 minutes.
5. Serve immediately.

Makes 4 servings

NUTRITIONAL INFORMATION PER SERVING

Calories 110	Carbohydrate 8g
Fat 4.5g	Fiber 1g
Cholesterol 0mg	Protein 10g

Miso

Miso has a salty, slightly sweet, and often nutty flavor. It is an ideal base for soup broths. Miso is a fermented bean paste and comes in a variety of flavors and colors. The 3 basic varieties of miso are developed by the injection of cooked soybeans with a mold (koji) cultivated in either barley, rice, or soybean base. The flavors and colors also differ depending on the length of time of the fermentation, generally between 6 months and 3 years. The darker miso varieties have been fermented for a longer period of time while the lighter, more delicately flavored miso has been fermented for a shorter period of time.

Miso pastes are available at Asian markets and most grocery stores. Dried paste in packets and paste in tubs are the most common forms. They are ready to eat and can be added to salad dressings, used as a soup base, or used to flavor marinades and sauces.

Kombu-Squash Soup

6 cups water

1 8-inch piece kombu

4 cups chopped butternut squash

1 tablespoon extra-virgin olive oil

1 large yellow onion, chopped

4 cloves garlic, minced

1 2-inch piece fresh gingerroot, chopped

¼ cup soy sauce or tamari

1. Bring the water to a boil in a large saucepan. Add the kombu and squash and cook over medium heat for 20 minutes.

2. Remove the kombu from the pot and spread the fronds out on a cutting board. Cut the tough spine from the kombu with a knife. Discard the spine and return the soft sheets of kombu to the saucepan.

3. Remove the squash from the pot and cut away the skin. Discard the skin and return the squash to the pot.

4. Heat the olive oil in a skillet. Add the onion, garlic, and ginger and sauté for 10 minutes.
5. Add the sautéed vegetables to the pot with the squash and kombu and cook for 1 hour.
6. Add soy sauce or tamari and serve.

⌒ Makes 10 servings

Kombu

This popular sea vegetable, also known as kelp, is one of the basic ingredients used in Japanese soup stocks. The long, dark brown seaweed is harvested from the ocean, folded into sheets, and sun-dried.

Kombu is sold in Asian markets and health-food stores and when stored unopened in a dry place it will keep indefinitely. After opening, store in a cool, dry place up to 6 months.

NUTRITIONAL INFORMATION PER SERVING

Calories 60	Carbohydrate 11g
Fat 1.5g	Fiber 3g
Cholesterol 0mg	Protein 1g

Chinese Cabbage and Dulse Soup

....

5 cups water
1 8-inch piece dulse
1 cup finely chopped carrot
4 cups finely chopped cabbage
1 yellow onion, chopped
¼ cup tamari or soy sauce

1. Place all ingredients in a large saucepan and heat over medium heat until boiling.
2. Reduce heat and simmer for 15 minutes.
3. Serve hot.

Makes 4 servings

NUTRITIONAL INFORMATION PER SERVING

Calories 80	Carbohydrate 14g
Fat 0.5g	Fiber 3g
Cholesterol 0mg	Protein 5g

Gazpacho

....

1 cup finely chopped red onion

2 cups finely chopped cucumber

1 cup diced green bell pepper

1 cup finely chopped red bell pepper

3 cloves garlic, minced

¼ jalapeño pepper, minced

1 cup finely chopped cilantro

1 28-ounce can tomato puree

¼ cup rice vinegar

¼ cup dry red wine or balsamic vinegar

¼ cup water

1 tablespoon fresh lime juice

3 tablespoons fresh lemon juice

½ teaspoon freshly ground black pepper

1. Combine all ingredients in a large container.
2. Chill for at least 20 minutes. This cold soup can be refrigerated in an airtight container for up to 5 days.
3. Serve chilled.

Makes 8 servings

NUTRITIONAL INFORMATION PER SERVING

Calories 100

Fat 1g

Cholesterol omg

Carbohydrate 15g

Fiber 3g

Protein 8g

Spicy Japanese Broth

1½ pounds firm tofu, cubed
3 cups vegetable broth
4 tablespoons tamari or soy sauce
2 tablespoons mirin
1 2-inch piece fresh gingerroot, pressed
¼ cup sliced scallions
½ cup thinly sliced canned bamboo shoots

1. Combine all ingredients in a saucepan and heat gently over medium heat.
2. Serve hot.

Makes 8 servings

NUTRITIONAL INFORMATION PER SERVING

Calories 100	Carbohydrate 5g
Fat 4.5g	Fiber 1g
Cholesterol omg	Protein 9g

Herbed Soup

10 cloves garlic, minced
½ cup chopped fresh Italian parsley or cilantro
2 bay leaves
1 teaspoon dried sage
5 whole cloves
Pinch of crushed dried thyme
2 quarts vegetable broth
¼ teaspoon freshly ground black pepper
3 tablespoons tamari or soy sauce
1 14-ounce can stewed tomatoes
3 tablespoons fresh lemon juice
1 1-pound can cooked white beans
Pinch of saffron threads

1. Place all ingredients except the saffron in a large stock-pot and bring to a boil. Stir well, cover, reduce heat, and simmer for 30 minutes.
2. While the soup is cooking, dry-roast the saffron: heat a skillet over low heat. Add the saffron and cook gently, stirring constantly for 3 minutes to release the oils.
3. Add the saffron to the soup, remove from heat, and let sit for 5 minutes.
4. Serve warm.

Makes 8 servings

NUTRITIONAL INFORMATION PER SERVING

Calories 110	Carbohydrate 18g
Fat 1.5g	Fiber 4g
Cholesterol 0mg	Protein 7g

Creamy Chinese Soup

2 cups plain soy milk
1 quart vegetable broth
1½ teaspoons tamari or soy sauce
¼ teaspoon salt
6 ounces firm tofu, cubed
1½ teaspoons sesame oil
½ Chinese cabbage, sliced
½ cup bean sprouts
1 teaspoon minced fresh gingerroot
3 tablespoons minced fresh parsley

1. Place all ingredients in a saucepan and heat gently.
2. Serve hot.

Makes 8 servings

NUTRITIONAL INFORMATION PER SERVING

Calories 80	Carbohydrate 11g
Fat 2.5g	Fiber 0g
Cholesterol 0mg	Protein 5g

Baked Herb Fries

1 large russet potato
1 teaspoon extra-virgin olive oil
¼ teaspoon crushed dried rosemary
¼ teaspoon crushed dried basil
½ teaspoon mild paprika
1 teaspoon sea salt

1. Preheat the oven to 450°F.
2. Slice the potato into long thin strips
3. Combine all ingredients in a large bowl. Toss until the potatoes are well coated with oil and seasonings.
4. Spread onto a baking sheet and bake for 15 minutes. Remove from oven and turn potatoes over. Bake for 15 more minutes, or until golden brown.
5. Serve with Tofu Ketchup (see Index).

Makes 2 servings

NUTRITIONAL INFORMATION PER SERVING

Calories 130	Carbohydrate 26g
Fat 2.5g	Fiber 2g
Cholesterol 0mg	Protein 2g

Spiced Cream of Pumpkin Soup

1 cup pumpkin seeds
1 tablespoon extra-virgin olive oil
3 large leeks, cleaned and chopped
½ pound carrots, sliced thin
3 cups vegetable broth
1 15-ounce can solid-pack pumpkin
2 cups nonfat milk or soy milk
¼ teaspoon ground nutmeg
¼ teaspoon ground cinnamon

1. Heat a skillet over high heat. Add the pumpkin seeds and toast, stirring constantly, until they puff up. Remove from heat and set aside.
2. Place the olive oil in the skillet over medium heat. Add the leeks and carrot and sauté until leeks are browned.

3. Add 2 cups of the broth and simmer for about 10 minutes.
4. Remove the leeks, carrots, and broth to a blender and process until creamy. Return to the pan and add the remaining broth, pumpkin, milk, nutmeg, and cinnamon. Cover and simmer for 15 minutes, stirring often, until hot.
5. Pour into serving bowls and sprinkle each bowl with 1 tablespoon toasted pumpkin seeds.

⌇ Makes 4 servings

NUTRITIONAL INFORMATION PER SERVING

Calories 430	Carbohydrate 46g
Fat 20g	Fiber 8g
Cholesterol 0mg	Protein 17g

Baked Beans

....

1 tablespoon extra-virgin olive oil

½ yellow onion, chopped

3 cloves garlic, chopped

2 cups cooked adzuki, kidney, or pinto beans

1 tablespoon molasses

1 tablespoon tamari or soy sauce

1 teaspoon dry mustard

1 tablespoon canola oil

1. Preheat the oven to 350°F.
2. Heat the olive oil in a large skillet. Add the onion and garlic and sauté over medium heat until the onion is translucent. Add the beans, molasses, tamari, and mustard. Stir well.
3. Oil a baking dish with the canola oil and add the bean mixture. Bake for 20 minutes or until golden brown.

Makes 4 servings

NUTRITIONAL INFORMATION PER SERVING

Calories 240	Carbohydrate 35g
Fat 7g	Fiber 1g
Cholesterol 0mg	Protein 9g

White Bean and Green Herb Salad

3 cups cooked white beans

4 fresh ripe Roma tomatoes, chopped

½ red onion, sliced into thin slivers

3 cloves garlic, diced

1 teaspoon chopped fresh thyme

¼ cup chopped fresh Italian parsley leaves

¼ cup chopped fresh basil leaves

¼ cup grated Parmesan or soy Parmesan cheese

1 tablespoon extra-virgin olive oil

¼ to ½ teaspoon hot red pepper flakes

Pinch of sea salt

¼ teaspoon black pepper

1. Place all ingredients in a large bowl and toss together until mixed well.
2. Serve chilled or at room temperature.

Makes 4 servings

NUTRITIONAL INFORMATION PER SERVING

Calories 290	Carbohydrate 43g
Fat 6g	Fiber 11g
Cholesterol 5mg	Protein 17g

Hijiki and Shiitake Mushrooms

....

1 cup hijiki
4 shiitake mushrooms, stemmed and sliced
3 tablespoons tamari or soy sauce
1 tablespoon sesame oil

1. Rinse the hijiki. Soak it in ½ cup water for 10 minutes, then drain (reserving the soaking water) and slice thin.
2. Place the hijiki and mushrooms in a saucepan with the soaking water and bring to a boil. Reduce heat and simmer for 40 to 45 minutes, or until hijiki is very soft. (If necessary, add more water.)
3. Season with tamari and sesame oil and serve.

∼ Makes 2 servings

NUTRITIONAL INFORMATION PER SERVING

Calories 70	Carbohydrate 10g
Fat 2.5g	Fiber 6g
Cholesterol 0mg	Protein 2g

Spicy Corn Bread

....

1 cup whole wheat pastry flour
1 cup cornmeal
½ teaspoon freshly ground sea salt
1 egg white
1 large egg
1 cup cold water
½ cup fresh corn kernels
1 jalapeño pepper, minced
¼ cup grated soy Parmesan or low-fat cheddar cheese

1. Preheat the oven to 400°F.
2. Mix together the flour, cornmeal, and salt in a medium bowl.
3. In a separate bowl, whip together the egg white, egg, and water. Fold the dry ingredients into the liquid; add the corn, jalapeño, and cheese; and mix together.
4. Pour the batter into a nonstick 9 × 5 × 3-inch baking dish. Bake for 20 to 25 minutes, or until golden brown.

⁓ *Makes 6 servings*

NUTRITIONAL INFORMATION PER SERVING

Calories 210	Carbohydrate 38g
Fat 3g	Fiber 5g
Cholesterol 40mg	Protein 8g

Roasted Eggplant and Mozzarella Sandwich

....

2 large firm eggplants
8 slices whole wheat bread
1 teaspoon mild paprika
1 tablespoon Dijon mustard
2 large fresh ripe tomatoes, sliced
¼ pound mozzarella cheese, grated

1. Preheat the oven to 400°F.
2. Roast the eggplants in the oven until the skins puff up. Let cool, then remove the skins with a knife. Cut the eggplant flesh into ½-inch slices.
3. Toast the bread. Mix the paprika and mustard together and spread on toast.
4. Place tomatoes, eggplant, and grated cheese on each slice.
5. Serve warm.

Makes 8 servings

NUTRITIONAL INFORMATION PER SERVING

Calories 140	Carbohydrate 20g
Fat 3.5g	Fiber 4g
Cholesterol 10mg	Protein 7g

Creamy Tomato Pasta

6 ounces silken tofu

12 ounces prepared marinara sauce

½ cup chopped Italian parsley

¼ teaspoon crushed dried oregano

¼ teaspoon crushed dried basil

¼ teaspoon crushed dried thyme

1 cup whole-grain pasta

4 tablespoons grated soy Parmesan cheese

1. Place the tofu and marinara sauce in a blender and process until smooth. Add the herbs and mix well.
2. Place the sauce in a saucepan and heat over low heat just until hot.
3. Cook the pasta according to package directions. Drain.
4. Divide the pasta among 4 bowls and top each portion with ½ cup sauce and 1 tablespoon soy Parmesan cheese.

∼ Makes 4 servings

NUTRITIONAL INFORMATION PER SERVING

Calories 220	Carbohydrate 32g
Fat 5g	Fiber 4g
Cholesterol 5mg	Protein 11g

Lentil Stew

....

2 cups water

1 cup lentils, rinsed

1 4-inch piece kombu (optional)

1 tablespoon extra-virgin olive oil

1 large carrot, julienned

1 large yellow onion, chopped

3 cloves garlic, crushed

1 14-ounce can Italian tomatoes

4 teaspoons ground cumin

½ teaspoon coriander

½ teaspoon sea salt

¼ teaspoon black pepper

2 tablespoons balsamic vinegar

1. Cook lentils (and kombu, if desired) in water for 20 minutes.
2. Sauté carrot, onion, and garlic in olive oil for 10 minutes in a large skillet.
3. Add lentils, tomatoes, cumin, coriander, salt, pepper, and vinegar and cook an additional 15 minutes on low heat.
4. Serve hot.

~ Makes 4 servings

NUTRITIONAL INFORMATION PER SERVING

Calories 260	Carbohydrate 45g
Fat 3.5g	Fiber 6g
Cholesterol 0mg	Protein 13g

Spicy Quinoa Pilaf with Fish

2 cups water

1 cup quinoa, rinsed well to remove any debris

1 tablespoon extra-virgin olive oil

½ cup finely chopped sweet onion

½ cup finely chopped red bell pepper

½ cup finely chopped yellow bell pepper

½ cup chopped cilantro

¼ teaspoon freshly ground sea salt

6 filets of a light, flaky fish, such as sole, halibut, or flounder

1½ cups hot salsa (without oils or sugars)

1. Bring the water to a boil and add the quinoa. Reduce heat and simmer for 10 minutes.
2. Heat the oil in a skillet. Add the onion, peppers, cilantro, and salt and cook over medium heat until the onion becomes translucent, about 5 minutes.
3. Place the fish on top of the vegetables, cover and heat for 10 minutes to cook the fish.
4. Serve the vegetables and fish over the quinoa with salsa on the side.

⤳ Makes 6 servings

NUTRITIONAL INFORMATION PER SERVING

Calories 443	Carbohydrate 42g
Fat 17g	Fiber 5g
Cholesterol 69mg	Protein 35g

3

Snacks and Beverages

Edamame

....

1 pound organic green soybeans (shelled)
Sea salt

1. Steam the soybeans in a bamboo steamer or in a saucepan
   with a mesh steamer basket for 5 to 8 minutes.
2. Salt to taste and serve hot.

~℃ *Makes 4 servings*

*Note: For quickly steaming vegetables, a bamboo steamer is ideal.
It fits over a saucepan, skillet, or wok and needs only a rinse to clean.
Bamboo steamers can be purchased at most natural-food markets and
health-food stores and at many shops selling kitchen appliances.*

*Young green soybeans are generally sold in their pods or without
pods in plastic bags in the freezer department of natural-food stores
or Asian markets.*

NUTRITIONAL INFORMATION PER SERVING

Calories 160	Carbohydrate 13g
Fat 7g	Fiber 5g
Cholesterol 0mg	Protein 14g

Arame with Onions

....

1 ounce dried arame
1 tablespoon toasted sesame oil
2 yellow onions, sliced
2 tablespoons water
3 tablespoons tamari or soy sauce
2 tablespoons toasted sesame seeds

1. Wash and drain the arame.
2. Heat the oil in a medium skillet, then add the onions and cook for 2 to 3 minutes.
3. Add the arame and water and bring to a boil, then reduce heat to low. Add the tamari, cover, and simmer for 40 to 50 minutes.
4. Remove from heat. Add more tamari, if desired, and sprinkle with sesame seeds.
5. Serve warm or cold.

Makes 4 servings

NUTRITIONAL INFORMATION PER SERVING

Calories 100	Carbohydrate 10g
Fat 6g	Fiber 2g
Cholesterol 0mg	Protein 2g

Toasted Nori Squares

....

4 sheets nori
2 tablespoons freshly grated gingerroot
2 tablespoons tamari or soy sauce
2 tablespoons mirin

1. Toast the sheets of nori for a few seconds each (either over the flame of a gas stove or the hot element of an electric stove). When the nori becomes dry and crisp, cut the sheets into 2-inch squares and place several squares of nori on a serving plate.
2. Place a pinch of grated ginger and 2 to 3 drops of tamari and mirin on each.
3. Fold up the nori with the ginger and sauce inside.

Makes 4 servings

NUTRITIONAL INFORMATION PER SERVING

Calories 35	Carbohydrate 7g
Fat 0g	Fiber 1g
Cholesterol 0mg	Protein 1g

Popcorn

....

1 tablespoon popcorn kernels
3 tablespoons nutritional yeast flakes

1. Use a hot-air popcorn machine to eliminate need for oil.
2. Place the freshly popped popcorn into a paper bag. Pour the nutritional yeast flakes into the bag while the popcorn is still warm so that the steam will help the yeast stick to the popcorn. Close up the bag and shake to coat the popcorn evenly.
3. Serve immediately.

⌁ Makes 1 serving

NUTRITIONAL INFORMATION PER SERVING

Calories 150	Carbohydrate 23g
Fat 1g	Fiber 11g
Cholesterol 0mg	Protein 13g

Soy Yogurt and Apricots

½ cup fresh organic apricots, pitted
½ cup plain, nonfat organic soy yogurt

1. Cut the apricots in half or chop.
2. Mix into the soy yogurt.
3. Serve chilled.

~ Makes 1 serving

NUTRITIONAL INFORMATION PER SERVING

Calories 150	Carbohydrate 21g
Fat 4g	Fiber 5g
Cholesterol 0mg	Protein 8g

Strawberry Squares

1 quart fresh organic strawberries
2 tablespoons agar flakes

1. Puree the strawberries in a blender.
2. Place the strawberry puree in a saucepan and heat gently. Add the agar flakes to the puree and continue to heat until the flakes have dissolved.
3. Pour the puree into a shallow, wide-bottomed pan and place in the refrigerator. As the puree cools, it will gel.
4. When well gelled, cut into cubes.
5. Serve cold.

Makes 6 servings

NUTRITIONAL INFORMATION PER SERVING

Calories 70	Carbohydrate 16g
Fat 0g	Fiber 5g
Cholesterol 0mg	Protein 1g

Banana Smoothie

....

½ frozen banana

1 cup plain soy milk

1 teaspoon barley malt syrup

1. Freeze the banana ahead of time by peeling it and placing it into a plastic bag in the freezer. Do not freeze with
   the peel intact; it is very difficult to remove once frozen.
2. Place the frozen banana, soy milk, and syrup into a
   blender and process just until smooth.
3. Serve immediately.

⌒ Makes 1 serving

NUTRITIONAL INFORMATION PER SERVING

Calories 200	Carbohydrate 37g
Fat 3g	Fiber 1g
Cholesterol 0mg	Protein 9g

Raspberry Vanilla Smoothie

6 ounces plain nonfat yogurt
½ cup frozen raspberries
½ cup silken tofu
1 teaspoon vanilla extract

1. Place all ingredients in a blender and process until smooth.
2. Drink immediately.

Makes 2 servings

NUTRITIONAL INFORMATION PER SERVING

Calories 70	Carbohydrate 11 g
Fat 0 g	Fiber 2 g
Cholesterol 0 mg	Protein 5 g

Licorice Smoothie

....

1 cup plain nonfat yogurt (frozen)
1 cup plain soy milk
1 teaspoon licorice root extract
6 ounces silken tofu

1. Place the yogurt in the freezer for at least 1 hour prior to blending.
2. Place all ingredients in a blender and puree until smooth and creamy.
2. Drink immediately.

Makes 2 servings

NUTRITIONAL INFORMATION PER SERVING

Calories 166	Carbohydrate 19g
Fat 3g	Fiber 0g
Cholesterol 2mg	Protein 17g

Vanilla Licorice Shake

1 frozen banana
½ cup plain nonfat yogurt
½ cup silken tofu
1 tablespoon ground flaxseed
1 teaspoon licorice root extract
1 teaspoon vanilla extract

1. Freeze the banana ahead of time by peeling it and placing it in a plastic bag in the freezer. Do not freeze with the peel intact; it is very difficult to remove once frozen.
2. Place all ingredients in a blender and puree until smooth.
3. Drink immediately.

Makes 2 servings

NUTRITIONAL INFORMATION PER SERVING

Calories 150

Fat 3.5g

Cholesterol 0mg

Carbohydrate 22g

Fiber 3g

Protein 8g

Chocolate Banana
Milk Shake

....

1 cup nonfat soy milk

1 drop stevia liquid extract

¼ teaspoon guar gum

1 frozen banana

2 teaspoons unsweetened chocolate powder

4 ice cubes

1. Place all ingredients in a blender and process until smooth.
2. Serve immediately.

Makes 2 servings

Health Benefits of Stevia

Although stevia has traditionally been used as a sweetener, studies have shown that stevia also has mild antibacterial properties. It has also been shown to inhibit the development of plaque and aid in the prevention of dental caries.

NUTRITIONAL INFORMATION PER SERVING

Calories 100	Carbohydrate 19g
Fat 0g	Fiber 1g
Cholesterol 0mg	Protein 5g

Carob Cocoa

....

1 cup plain or vanilla soy milk
1 teaspoon organic turbinado sugar
1 tablespoon unsweetened carob powder

1. Heat the soy milk in a saucepan or in a mug in the microwave.
2. Dissolve the sugar into the milk and add the carob powder. Mix well.
3. Serve immediately.

∽ Makes 1 serving

NUTRITIONAL INFORMATION PER SERVING

Calories 90	Carbohydrate 8g
Fat 3.5g	Fiber 2g
Cholesterol 0mg	Protein 6g

Licorice Root Tea

¼ teaspoon licorice root extract
1 cup boiling water

1. Dissolve the thick licorice paste into the hot water.
2. Drink immediately.

Makes 1 serving

Licorice Root

Licorice (glycyrrhiza glabra) is sold as a dried root, liquid extract, or powder extract. Licorice tea bags are sold at natural-food markets. Drinking tea made from the extract of licorice is known to relieve the symptoms of menopause, help fight infections and illness caused by virus, and reduce the inflammation associated with arthritis. The sale of the liquid extract is regulated because extensive consumption can lead to an increase in blood pressure in some people. It must be purchased through a nutritionist or a naturopathic doctor.

NUTRITIONAL INFORMATION PER SERVING

Calories 5	Carbohydrate 1g
Fat 0g	Fiber 0g
Cholesterol 0mg	Protein 0g

Green Tea

....

1 caffeine-free green tea bag
1 cup boiling water

1. Steep the tea bag in the hot water for about 5 minutes.
2. Drink immediately.

~ *Makes 1 serving*

Green Tea

Studies have shown that green tea (camellia sinensis) has the ability, when taken in extract form, to significantly reduce blood glucose levels in diabetics. It has been found to have both preventive and curative effects on diabetic rats.

NUTRITIONAL INFORMATION PER SERVING

Calories 0	Carbohydrate 0g
Fat 0g	Fiber 0g
Cholesterol 0mg	Protein 0g

Fenugreek Tea

....

1 teaspoon fenugreek seeds
1 cup water

1. Mix the fenugreek seeds into the water and soak overnight.
2. In the morning, boil the seeds and water. Strain the seeds out.
3. Drink the remaining tea hot.

Makes 1 serving

Fenugreek

Fenugreek (trigonella foenumgraecum) seeds are sold as a spice or can be purchased in the produce department of the grocery store. The seeds may be eaten raw to reduce fasting blood sugar and improve glucose tolerance.

NUTRITIONAL INFORMATION PER SERVING

Calories 15	Carbohydrate 2g
Fat 0g	Fiber 1g
Cholesterol 0mg	Protein 1g

4

Dinner

Nori Rolls

¼ cup grated cucumber
Dash of tamari or soy sauce
1 teaspoon toasted sesame seeds
1 cup cooked crabmeat
2 tablespoons rice vinegar
½ teaspoon kelp powder
2 cups hot cooked brown rice
4 sheets toasted nori

1. Mix together the cucumber, tamari, sesame seeds, and crabmeat in a bowl and set aside.
2. In a separate bowl, mix together the vinegar, kelp, and hot rice.
3. Place a sheet of nori on a small bamboo mat or heavy cloth napkin. Spread ½ cup of rice mixture over the sheet and arrange ¼ of the cucumber-crabmeat filling in a line across the middle of the rice. Roll up the nori on the mat, wetting the end to stick the roll together. Repeat with remaining nori sheets.
4. Slice into 1-inch rolls.

Makes 4 servings

NUTRITIONAL INFORMATION PER SERVING

Calories 160	Carbohydrate 24g
Fat 2g	Fiber 3g
Cholesterol 35mg	Protein 10g

Coleslaw

....

3 cups thinly sliced cabbage

1 cup thinly sliced carrot

1 tablespoon finely chopped yellow onion

1 teaspoon minced fresh Italian parsley

3 tablespoons Dijon mustard

1 tablespoon rice vinegar

1 tablespoon balsamic vinegar

¼ cup plain nonfat yogurt or tofu mayonnaise

½ teaspoon honey

½ teaspoon sea salt

2 teaspoons caraway seeds

¼ teaspoon freshly ground black pepper

¼ teaspoon celery seed

1. Place all ingredients in a large bowl and mix together thoroughly.
2. Serve chilled. This salad can be stored in an airtight container in the refrigerator for up to 4 days.

~ *Makes 6 servings*

NUTRITIONAL INFORMATION PER SERVING

Calories 25

Fat 0g

Cholesterol 0mg

Carbohydrate 5g

Fiber 1g

Protein 1g

Bitter Melon Stir-Fry

....

1 teaspoon extra-virgin olive oil
¼ pound fresh snow peas
1 tablespoon freshly grated gingerroot
1 bitter melon, sliced thin
1 red pear, cored and sliced thin

1. Heat the olive oil in a skillet.
2. Add the snow peas and ginger and sauté for 5 minutes. Add the bitter melon and cook over medium heat for another 5 minutes. Add the pear and cook for 3 minutes longer.
3. Serve warm.

Makes 4 servings

Bitter Melon

Bitter melon is also known as balsam pear, bitter cucumber, foogwa, la kwa, *and, in Indian languages,* karela. *It comes from China, Hong Kong, the Philippines, Taiwan, and India. It is available in many natural-food markets and grocery stores in the United States and Canada. Studies of bitter melon show blood-sugar-lowering and regulating effects when eaten raw or cooked. Use this vegetable in stir-fry, stews, and soups.*

NUTRITIONAL INFORMATION PER SERVING

Calories 60	Carbohydrate 11g
Fat 1.5g	Fiber 3g
Cholesterol 0mg	Protein 2g

Sautéed Hijiki

....

1 cup hijiki

2 cups water

2 tablespoons toasted sesame oil

1. Soak the hijiki in 2 cups water for 10 minutes. (Hijiki will be soft.) Drain and chop.
2. Heat the oil in a skillet over medium heat. Add the hijiki and sauté for 2 minutes.
3. Serve hot.

∼ Makes 2 servings

NUTRITIONAL INFORMATION PER SERVING

Calories 150	Carbohydrate 6g
Fat 14g	Fiber 6g
Cholesterol 0mg	Protein 0g

Arame-Stuffed Mushrooms

1 cup chopped dried arame

1½ cups vegetable broth

1 pound large mushrooms

1 tablespoon extra-virgin olive oil

½ yellow onion, minced

5 cloves garlic, minced

¼ cup tamari or soy sauce

⅛ teaspoon cayenne

1 teaspoon dried Italian seasoning *or* 2 tablespoons minced
fresh basil, oregano, sage, or thyme

½ cup dry bread crumbs

½ cup grated Parmesan or soy Parmesan cheese

1. Preheat the oven to 350°F.
2. Soak the chopped arame in the vegetable broth for 10 minutes to reconstitute. Remove the stems from the mushrooms, reserving the caps for stuffing. Dice the stems.
3. Heat the olive oil in a skillet. Add the chopped mushroom stems, onion, and garlic and sauté for 5 minutes.

4. Place the reconstituted arame and about 1 cup of the broth it has been soaking in into a blender. Add the tamari, cayenne, and spices and blend well.

5. Remove the arame from the blender into a bowl. Add the remaining soaking liquid and the sautéed mixture, then add the bread crumbs. Stuff the mushroom caps with the mixture and sprinkle with Parmesan cheese. Bake for 15 to 20 minutes.

6. Serve hot.

~ *Makes 4 servings*

NUTRITIONAL INFORMATION PER SERVING

Calories 220	Carbohydrate 27g
Fat 8g	Fiber 5g
Cholesterol 15mg	Protein 11g

Asian Kombu Potato Sauté

....

1 12-inch piece kombu
1 tablespoon extra-virgin olive oil
1 sweet potato, chopped
1 russet potato, chopped
1 red potato, chopped
1 yellow onion, chopped
½ cup water
3 tablespoons balsamic vinegar
2 tablespoons tamari or soy sauce

1. Soak the kombu in 2 cups water until soft, about 10 minutes. Drain. Cut out the tough spine and chop the soft flesh.
2. Heat the olive oil in a large skillet. Add the potatoes, onion, and kombu and sauté over medium heat until golden brown.
3. Add the water, vinegar, and soy sauce; stir; and simmer for 5 minutes.
4. Serve hot.

~ *Makes 4 servings*

NUTRITIONAL INFORMATION PER SERVING

Calories 140	Carbohydrate 22g
Fat 4.5g	Fiber 2g
Cholesterol 0mg	Protein 2g

Baked Root Vegetables

2 sweet potatoes, chopped

1 russet potato, chopped

2 carrots, chopped

10 to 20 cloves garlic, peeled

3 tablespoons soy sauce or tamari

1 tablespoon extra-virgin olive oil

Salsa for topping (optional)

1. Preheat the oven to 350°F.
2. Toss all ingredients except salsa together in a large bowl until the vegetables are coated with oil and soy sauce.
3. Place the vegetables on a baking sheet and bake for 25 minutes, until vegetables are golden brown.
4. Serve with salsa, if desired.

Makes 6 servings

Note: All of these vegetables are high in chromium, which is an essential nutrient for proper blood-sugar metabolism.

NUTRITIONAL INFORMATION PER SERVING

Calories 140	Carbohydrate 26g
Fat 2.5g	Fiber 3g
Cholesterol 0mg	Protein 3g

Baked Potatoes with Onion Sauce

4 russet potatoes
¼ teaspoon toasted sesame oil
2 large sweet onions, diced
1 cup vegetable broth
¼ cup balsamic vinegar
1 tablespoon soy sauce or tamari
1 tablespoon arrowroot powder
2 tablespoons red wine

1. Preheat the oven to 350°F.
2. Poke the potatoes with a fork, place in oven, and bake for 45–60 minutes.
3. Heat the sesame oil in a skillet over medium heat. Add the onions and sauté over medium heat until browned.
4. Add the broth, vinegar, and tamari and simmer for 5 minutes. Remove from heat.
5. Mix the arrowroot into the red wine to liquefy, then stir into the onion sauce.
6. Serve the sauce over the baked potatoes.

Makes 4 servings

NUTRITIONAL INFORMATION PER SERVING

Calories 280	Carbohydrate 62g
Fat 0.5g	Fiber 6g
Cholesterol 0mg	Protein 6g

Tofu-Stuffed Manicotti

8 manicotti noodles

1 pound firm tofu, crumbled

1 teaspoon crushed dried oregano

1 teaspoon crushed dried thyme

1 teaspoon crushed dried basil

3 cloves garlic, minced

½ cup minced fresh Italian parsley

1 16-ounce jar prepared marinara sauce

1. Preheat the oven to 375°F. Cook the noodles according to package instructions, drain, and set aside.
2. In a large bowl, combine the tofu, herbs, garlic, and parsley. Stuff the manicotti with the tofu filling.
3. Place the stuffed noodles in an 8-inch square baking dish, pour the marinara sauce over the manicotti, and bake for 30 minutes.
4. Serve hot.

Makes 4 servings

NUTRITIONAL INFORMATION PER SERVING

Calories 240	Carbohydrate 29g
Fat 8g	Fiber 0g
Cholesterol 20mg	Protein 13g

Vegetable Curry

....

2 teaspoons black mustard seeds

2 teaspoons cumin seeds

1 cup fresh green peas

1 cup diced potato

2 cups fresh green beans

1 cup diced carrot

2 teaspoons turmeric

1½ cups water

½ cup plain nonfat yogurt

2 tablespoons flaxseed oil

1 teaspoon sea salt

1 teaspoon coriander powder

1. Roast the mustard and cumin seeds in a dry skillet over high heat.
2. When the seeds begin to pop, add the peas, potatoes, green beans, carrots, turmeric, and water. Stir well, then cover and cook for 15 to 20 minutes.
3. Add the yogurt, oil, salt, and coriander, stirring well. Cover again and simmer on low heat for another 15 to 20 minutes.
4. Serve hot.

Makes 6 servings

NUTRITIONAL INFORMATION PER SERVING

Calories 140

Fat 6g

Cholesterol 0mg

Carbohydrate 17g

Fiber 4g

Protein 5g

Fish and Eggplant Curry

1½ teaspoons extra-virgin olive oil
3 cups chopped eggplant
1 cup chopped yellow onion
2 cups sliced mushrooms
2 tablespoons red curry paste
1 cup reduced fat coconut milk
1 pound fish (such as cod or halibut)
1 cup cooked brown rice

1. Heat the olive oil in a large skillet over medium heat. Add the eggplant, onion, and mushrooms and cook for 5 minutes stirring occasionally. Stir in the curry paste.
2. Pour in the coconut milk. Place the fish on top and cook for another 10 minutes, turning the fish as needed until it is thoroughly cooked.
3. Break up the fish and mix it into the sauce.
4. Distribute the rice evenly onto 4 serving plates and pour equal amounts of curry sauce over each dish.

Makes 4 servings

NUTRITIONAL INFORMATION PER SERVING

Calories 329	Carbohydrate 32g
Fat 10g	Fiber 5g
Cholesterol 36mg	Protein 28g

Herbed Fish with Spicy Salsa

SALSA

4 large fresh ripe tomatoes, chopped
¼ cup chopped red onion
1 cup chopped cilantro
3 cloves garlic, chopped
¼ jalapeño pepper, chopped
1 teaspoon chopped fresh oregano *or* a pinch of crushed dried
   oregano
¼ teaspoon freshly ground sea salt
Pinch of freshly ground black pepper

FISH

1 tablespoon toasted sesame oil
1 teaspoon mild paprika
1 teaspoon crushed dried thyme
1 teaspoon sea salt
1 clove garlic, pressed
6 6-ounce fillets flaky white fish

Directions for Salsa

1. Combine all ingredients in a large bowl and mix together
   thoroughly.
2. Set aside. (Salsa may be made in advance. Store in a covered container in the refrigerator for up to 5 days.)

Directions for Fish

1. In a mortar and pestle, grind together the oil, paprika, thyme, salt, and garlic until a smooth paste forms.
2. Rub the paste over the fish fillets.
3. Broil the fish in oven for about 7 minutes. (The cooking time will vary depending on the thickness of the fish fillets.)
4. When the fish is cooked thoroughly, pour salsa in equal amounts over each fish fillet.
5. Serve immediately.

~ *Makes 6 servings*

NUTRITIONAL INFORMATION PER SERVING

Calories 190	Carbohydrate 3g
Fat 4g	Fiber 1g
Cholesterol 85mg	Protein 36g

Marinated Tuna

¼ cup tamari or soy sauce

1 3-inch piece gingerroot, minced

4 cloves garlic, pressed

2 tablespoons balsamic vinegar

1 pound fresh tuna

1. Preheat the oven to 350°F.
2. Place the tamari, ginger, garlic, and vinegar in a large bowl and stir together.
3. Add the tuna, toss to coat, and marinate for at least 1 hour.
4. Place the fish on a baking dish and bake for 25 minutes, or until fish is flaky and brown.
5. Serve with Mango Salsa (see Index).

Makes 6 servings

> *Note: A well-designed garlic press eliminates the job of peeling and chopping garlic. When it's easier to prepare garlic for your recipes, you'll find that you use more of it.*

NUTRITIONAL INFORMATION PER SERVING

Calories 160	Carbohydrate 2g
Fat 6g	Fiber 0g
Cholesterol 15mg	Protein 23g

Blackened Catfish

2 catfish fillets
1 teaspoon black pepper
1 teaspoon crushed dried dill
Pinch of cayenne

1. Place the fish and spices in a resealable plastic bag. Gently blow up the bag and seal. Shake the fish until completely coated.
2. Place a skillet on the stove and heat until very hot. Remove the catfish from the bag and place in the hot skillet. Cover and cook for about 3 minutes per side, depending on the thickness of the fish.
3. Serve hot.

⌣ *Makes 2 servings*

Note: A cast-iron skillet is the best pan to use as it tolerates heat well.

NUTRITIONAL INFORMATION PER SERVING

Calories 130	Carbohydrate 0g
Fat 1.5g	Fiber 0g
Cholesterol 75mg	Protein 27g

Spicy Basil Chicken

2½ cups brown rice

2 tablespoons extra-virgin olive oil

10 cloves garlic, chopped finely

1 cup sliced onion

1 pound organic chicken breast, skinned and chopped

2 jalapeño peppers, cut into slivers

2 kaffir lime leaves, slivered

1 cup fresh holy basil, chopped

2 tablespoons tamari *or* soy sauce

1. Cook rice according to directions on package.
2. Heat the olive oil in a wok or large skillet. Add the garlic and onions and sauté for 2 minutes.
3. Add the chicken and cook for another 2 minutes.
4. Add the peppers, kaffir lime leaves, reconstituted holy basil, and tamari and continue to cook until chicken is no longer pink, about 10 minutes.
5. Distribute chicken and rice evenly onto 4 plates.
6. Serve hot.

Makes 4 servings

NUTRITIONAL INFORMATION PER SERVING

Calories 450	Carbohydrate 36g
Fat 17g	Fiber 3g
Cholesterol 95mg	Protein 38g

Lentil and Arame Stew

....

2 quarts vegetable broth

2 cups lentils, rinsed

¼ cup chopped arame

3 cloves garlic, minced

2 carrots, diced

1 stalk celery, diced

1 14-ounce can stewed tomatoes, drained and chopped

5 leaves fresh sage

1 bay leaf

1 teaspoon crushed dried oregano

Dash of cayenne (optional)

1. Place all ingredients in a saucepan and bring to a boil.
2. Reduce heat and simmer for 40 minutes, or until the lentils are tender.
3. Serve hot.

⌇ Makes 4 servings

NUTRITIONAL INFORMATION PER SERVING

Calories 450	Carbohydrate 86g
Fat 0g	Fiber 9g
Cholesterol 0mg	Protein 25g

Chicken and Pesto Dinner

2 cups fresh chopped holy basil leaves
¼ cup chopped walnuts
Juice of 1 lemon
4 cloves garlic
⅓ cup plain nonfat yogurt
½ cup freshly grated Parmesan cheese
½ cup chopped fresh Italian parsley
½ teaspoon freshly ground black pepper
½ teaspoon sea salt
1 pound organic chicken breasts, boneless
4 cups steamed vegetables (such as cabbage, broccoli, zucchini, or kale)

Directions for Pesto

1. In a large bowl combine holy basil (or common basil if you are unable to find holy basil), walnuts, lemon juice, garlic, yogurt, Parmesan cheese, Italian parsley, pepper, and salt.
2. Mix well and set aside.

Directions for Chicken and Vegetables

1. Preheat oven to 350 degrees.
2. Place chicken breasts in an oven-safe pan and bake for 25 minutes or until well cooked. (The cooking time will

vary depending on how thick the chicken breasts are. After cooking, use a knife to cut into the chicken breasts to be sure they are thoroughly cooked. If the meat in the middle is still pink or translucent, cook it longer. The meat will become a creamy-white color as it cooks.)

3. While the chicken is cooking, steam vegetables in a bamboo steamer or in a saucepan with 1 inch (2–4 cups depending on size of pan) of water over medium heat for about 5 minutes.

4. Cover and set aside.

5. Divide chicken and vegetables into 4 servings and place in individual bowls.

6. Pour the pesto sauce in equal portions over the chicken and vegetables in each dish.

7. Serve hot.

⌒ Makes 4 servings

NUTRITIONAL INFORMATION PER SERVING

Calories 460	Carbohydrate 16g
Fat 15g	Fiber 8g
Cholesterol 155mg	Protein 66g

Enchiladas and Red Sauce

Red Sauce

1 16-ounce can Roma tomatoes, drained

2 tablespoons chopped yellow onion

1 medium jalapeño pepper, chopped

3 cloves garlic, chopped

1 teaspoon ground cumin

1 teaspoon crushed dried oregano

1½ cups vegetable broth

Enchiladas

10 ounces firm tofu

1 14-ounce can black beans, drained

2 medium onions, diced

2 cloves garlic, minced

1 4-ounce can mild green chilies, drained and finely chopped

4 10-inch tortillas

8 ounces soy cheese (jack), grated

Directions for Red Sauce

1. Place tomatoes, onion, jalapeño, garlic, cumin, oregano, and broth in a blender or food processor and blend until well mixed.
2. Set aside.

Directions for Enchiladas

1. Combine the tofu, black beans, onions, garlic, and green chilies in a bowl.
2. Drop ¼ of the black bean combination into each tortilla and roll each one, tucking in the ends of each tortilla to secure the filling. Place these enchilada rolls in a baking dish and cover with red sauce.
3. Top with cheese.
4. Place in oven and bake for 20 minutes.
5. Serve hot.

Makes 4 servings

NUTRITIONAL INFORMATION PER SERVING

Calories 440	Carbohydrate 56g
Fat 12g	Fiber 16g
Cholesterol 0mg	Protein 28g

Herbed Cannellini

2 cups dried white beans, soaked overnight
6 cups water
2 16-ounce cans vegetable broth
1 cup chopped potato
1 head cabbage, sliced
1 cup sliced mushrooms
1 red bell pepper, sliced
1 teaspoon crushed dried thyme
1 teaspoon ground cumin
1 teaspoon crushed dried rosemary
2 bay leaves
2 tablespoons balsamic vinegar
2 tablespoons fresh lemon juice
1 tablespoon tamari or soy sauce
Salt
Black pepper

1. Drain the beans and place in a large saucepan. Add 6 cups fresh water, bring to a boil, cover, and simmer for 1 hour on low heat.
2. Add the broth and potato and cook for 10 more minutes.

3. Add the cabbage, mushrooms, bell pepper, herbs, vinegar, lemon juice, and soy sauce and cook for an additional 20 minutes.

4. Salt and pepper to taste. Serve hot.

Makes 4 servings

NUTRITIONAL INFORMATION PER SERVING

Calories 270	Carbohydrate 46g
Fat 2g	Fiber 10g
Cholesterol 0mg	Protein 17g

Black-Eyed Peas with Sun-Dried Tomatoes

3 cup black-eyed peas, soaked overnight

5 cups water

1 cup pearl barley

2 cups chopped yellow onion

5 sun-dried tomatoes, chopped

4 stalks celery, chopped

4 scallions, chopped

1 8-inch piece kombu, rib removed

4 carrots, chopped

2 cups chopped cilantro

2 tablespoons rice vinegar

2 teaspoons extra-virgin olive oil

2 teaspoons ground cumin

1. Drain the black-eyed peas and place in a saucepan with 5 cups fresh water. Bring to a boil, cover, and reduce heat, and simmer for 2 hours.
2. Add the barley and cook for 30 minutes more.
3. Add remaining ingredients and cook, covered, for 20 minutes.
4. Serve hot.

∼ Makes 2 servings

NUTRITIONAL INFORMATION PER SERVING

Calories 450	Carbohydrate 74g
Fat 8g	Fiber 23g
Cholesterol 0mg	Protein 20g

Tofu Meatballs

1 pound firm tofu, crumbled

2 large eggs

½ cup whole wheat bread crumbs

2 tablespoons tamari or soy sauce

½ teaspoon onion salt

½ teaspoon dried Italian seasoning

½ teaspoon garlic powder

¼ cup grated Parmesan cheese

1 tablespoon dried onion flakes

¼ teaspoon black pepper

¼ teaspoon ground nutmeg

1 tablespoon extra-virgin olive oil

1. Combine all ingredients except the olive oil in a large bowl. Mix well. Form into 1-inch balls.
2. Heat the oil in a large skillet and add the tofu balls. Sauté over medium-low heat until browned, turning often.
3. Serve with marinara sauce and pasta.

∼ Makes 8 servings

NUTRITIONAL INFORMATION PER SERVING

Calories 80	Carbohydrate 2g
Fat 5g	Fiber 0g
Cholesterol 55mg	Protein 7g

Beans, Greens, and Grains

....

This combination dish is a mainstay in my household. I learned to make this as a student because it is easy to cook up a pot of grain and a pot of beans ahead of time and have them in the fridge ready to go. I pick up fresh greens on the way home and throw together a nutrient-dense and delicious meal in just minutes.

    1 cup steamed greens
    ¼ cup cooked grain
    ½ cup cooked beans
    2 tablespoons dressing

Choose any combination of the following or add your favorites to the list. The greens in the chart that follows are particularly rich in minerals and vitamins. The vitamin-rich grains listed are high in fiber, and many of them, such as spelt, kamut, and quinoa, are higher in protein than wheat or rice. These beans are commonly available, but any beans can be used in this dish. These dressings are my favorites; see the Index for recipes.

GREENS	GRAIN	BEANS	SAUCE
Curly kale	Brown rice	Pinto	Ginger Dressing
Red kale	Barley	Kidney	Tahini
Swiss chard	Quinoa	Fava	Green Goddess Dressing
Spinach	Whole kernal rye	Black	Mango Salsa
Beet greens	Kamut	Garbanzo	Soy sauce or tamari
Mustard greens	Spelt	White	Balsamic vinegar

~ *Makes 1 serving*

Note: Nutritional amounts will vary slightly depending on which greens, grains, and beans you combine. This nutritional analysis is not based on dressing, but on greens, grains, and beans alone. Nutritional information is provided with the individual dressing recipes (see Index).

NUTRITIONAL INFORMATION PER SERVING

Calories 220	Carbohydrate 19g
Fat 1g	Fiber 8g
Cholesterol 0mg	Protein 13g

Marinated Tofu

....

1 tablespoon sesame oil

3 tablespoons crushed garlic

1 tablespoon minced fresh gingerroot

2 tablespoons soy sauce or tamari

1 tablespoon honey

1 pound firm tofu

1 tablespoon sesame seeds

1. Heat the sesame oil in a large skillet over medium heat. Add the garlic and ginger, and sauté for 2 minutes.
2. Stir in the tamari and honey until well mixed.
3. Slice the tofu into 8 slices and place carefully in the sauce.
4. Sauté the tofu over medium heat, browning each side.
5. Sprinkle with sesame seeds and serve warm with brown rice and miso soup.

∽ *Makes 8 servings*

NUTRITIONAL INFORMATION PER SERVING

Calories 70

Fat 4g

Cholesterol 0mg

Carbohydrate 4g

Fiber 0g

Protein 3g

5

Condiments

Tartar Sauce

¼ cup plain nonfat yogurt
¼ cup fat-free mayonnaise
¼ cup finely chopped pickle
¼ teaspoon dried dill
2 teaspoons fresh lemon juice

1. Mix all the ingredients together in a bowl until well blended.
2. Serve with fish or baked fries or mix with Tofu Ketchup (see Index) to make fry sauce.

~ *Makes 16 servings*

NUTRITIONAL INFORMATION PER SERVING

Calories 10	Carbohydrate 2g
Fat 0g	Fiber 0g
Cholesterol 0mg	Protein 0g

Tofu Ketchup

....

4 ounces silken tofu

1 tablespoon finely chopped yellow onion

2 cups tomato sauce

1 teaspoon extra-virgin olive oil

1 teaspoon fresh lemon juice

½ teaspoon unrefined cane sugar

1. Place all ingredients in a blender or food processor and process at medium speed until creamy.

Makes 33 servings

Note: Each serving is 1 heaping tablespoon.

NUTRITIONAL INFORMATION PER SERVING

Calories 15	Carbohydrate 1g
Fat 0g	Fiber 0g
Cholesterol 0mg	Protein 1g

Mango Salsa

....

1 mango, minced
½ cup chopped red bell pepper
½ cup minced red onion
1 tablespoon minced jalapeño pepper
1 tablespoon minced fresh mint leaves
1 tablespoon balsamic vinegar
2 tablespoons fresh lime juice
1 tomato, minced (optional)

1. Combined all ingredients in a medium bowl and mix thoroughly.
2. Serve immediately or store in a covered container in the refrigerator for up to 1 week.

Makes 6 servings

NUTRITIONAL INFORMATION PER SERVING

Calories 45   Carbohydrate 9g
Fat 0g   Fiber 2g
Cholesterol 0mg   Protein 1g

Kumquat Dressing

2 kumquats
½ lemon, peeled
1 tablespoon extra-virgin olive oil
2 tablespoons balsamic vinegar
1 tablespoon tamari or soy sauce
5 cloves garlic

1. Blend all ingredients together in a blender or food processor until smooth.
2. Serve over leafy greens or mixed green vegetables. (Dressing may be stored for up to 5 days in the refrigerator.)

~ *Makes 12 servings*

NUTRITIONAL INFORMATION PER SERVING

Calories 15	Carbohydrate 1g
Fat 1g	Fiber 0g
Cholesterol 0mg	Protein 0g

Ginger Dressing

½ orange
1 2-inch piece fresh gingerroot, peeled
5 cloves garlic
2 tablespoons soy sauce or tamari
2 tablespoons balsamic vinegar
1 tablespoon flaxseed oil or extra-virgin olive oil

1. Peel the orange by cutting off just the outside bright orange part of the peel, leaving the inner white pithy part, which contains all of its beneficial bioflavonoids.
2. Combine all ingredients in a blender and blend for 30 seconds to 1 minute. If you prefer a creamier dressing, blend longer. To thin the dressing add a tablespoon of water and blend again.
3. Serve over leafy greens or mixed dark-green vegetables.

Makes 16 servings

NUTRITIONAL INFORMATION PER SERVING

Calories 15	Carbohydrate 2g
Fat 1g	Fiber 0g
Cholesterol 0mg	Protein 0g

Garlic

Garlic (Allium sativum) contains sulphur compounds, which reduce the breakdown of insulin. This increases its availability, reducing blood-sugar levels. The medicinal compounds break down and become less potent when cooked, so raw is best. Add garlic to dips, salsa, fresh vegetable juices, or salad dressing.

Raw garlic is also a broad-spectrum antimicrobial. It is effective against staph, strep, bacillus, E. coli, salmonella, candida, roundworm, hookworm, and influenza. Garlic has potent cardiovascular benefits as well. Both raw and cooked garlic have been found to decrease triglyceride and cholesterol levels (total and ldl), raise hdl cholesterol, lower blood pressure, and prevent excessive blood-clot formation.

Asian Arame Dressing

2 tablespoons extra-virgin olive oil

2 tablespoons tamari or soy sauce

2 tablespoons balsamic vinegar

2 tablespoons fresh lemon juice

1 frond arame, reconstituted in water, drained

½ orange, peeled and seeded

1. Blend all ingredients together in a blender.
2. Serve dressing over salad, fish, beans, or grains.

~ Makes 6 servings

NUTRITIONAL INFORMATION PER SERVING

Calories 70	Carbohydrate 6g
Fat 4.5g	Fiber 3g
Cholesterol omg	Protein og

Green Goddess Salad Dressing

1 12.3-ounce package silken tofu
1 scallion, minced
½ cup minced fresh parsley
1 tablesoon fresh lemon juice
¼ teaspoon Dijon mustard
1 tablespoon extra-virgin olive oil
½ teaspoon sea salt

1. Combine all ingredients in a blender and blend until smooth.
2. Serve immediately (the ingredients tend to separate if left more than a few hours).

~ *Makes 18 servings*

NUTRITIONAL INFORMATION PER SERVING

Calories 20	Carbohydrate 1g
Fat 1g	Fiber 0g
Cholesterol 0mg	Protein 1g

Snow Peas with Wakame Dressing

....

1 tablespoon sesame oil

2 cups snow peas

12 ounces silken tofu, cubed

½ cup julienned carrot

4 large mushrooms, sliced

½ cup chopped wakame

1 tablespoon soy sauce or tamari

1 tablespoon tahini

1 tablespoon hot water

Juice of ½ lemon

Dash of ground nutmeg

Dash of cayenne

4 cups chopped fresh bok choy, Chinese cabbage, or greens

1. Heat the sesame oil in a large skillet.
2. Add the snow peas, tofu, carrots, mushrooms, and wakame and sauté for 5 minutes. Stir in the soy sauce.
3. Dissolve the tahini in the hot water; add the lemon juice, nutmeg, and cayenne; and pour over the sauté.
4. Serve warm over the bok choy, cabbage, or greens.

Makes 8 servings

NUTRITIONAL INFORMATION PER SERVING

Calories 120	Carbohydrate 11g
Fat 4g	Fiber 4g
Cholesterol 0mg	Protein 10g

Blackberry Jam

2 cups fresh blackberries
1½ teaspoons granulated agar

1. Place the berries in a blender and puree.
2. Pour the berry puree into a saucepan and sprinkle the agar on top. Let sit for 2 to 3 minutes until the agar has softened.
3. Bring to a simmer over low heat and stir until the agar dissolves, about 10 minutes.
4. Pour into serving dishes and chill in refrigerator until thickened.
5. Serve chilled on sandwiches with nut butter.

Makes 12 servings

NUTRITIONAL INFORMATION PER SERVING

Calories 20	Carbohydrate 5g
Fat 0g	Fiber 1g
Cholesterol 0mg	Protein 0g

Maple Syrup

....

¼ teaspoon guar gum

⅓ cup water

1 teaspoon maple flavoring

1 tablespoon pure maple syrup

Pinch of stevia extract powder *or* 3 drops stevia liquid
extract

¼ teaspoon hazelnut oil

1. Place all ingredients together in a blender and blend until
smooth.

2. Serve with pancakes or waffles.

~ *Makes 6 servings*

Stevia Sweetner

*Stevia is a safe, natural alternative to refined sugar and artificial
sweeteners. The Native Americans of Paraguay have used this herb for
centuries. Stevia is now available through health-food stores in the
United States and Canada.*

NUTRITIONAL INFORMATION PER SERVING

Calories 5	Carbohydrate 1g
Fat 0g	Fiber 0g
Cholesterol 0mg	Protein 0g

6

Desserts

Strawberry Pudding

....

1 ½ cups plain soy milk

2 cups ripe strawberries

1 teaspoon guar gum

2 teaspoons unrefined cane sugar

1 teaspoon vanilla extract and/or 1 tablespoon orange
juice concentrate (optional)

1. Place all ingredients in a blender and blend until smooth.
2. Pour into dessert dishes, cover tightly, and refrigerate for
   several hours.
3. Serve chilled.

Makes 8 servings

NUTRITIONAL INFORMATION PER SERVING

Calories 54	Carbohydrate 10g
Fat 1g	Fiber 1g
Cholesterol 0mg	Protein 2g

Chocolate Pudding

2 cups plain soy milk

3 tablespoons powdered unsweetened chocolate

2 teaspoons guar gum

4 tablespoons unrefined cane sugar

2 teaspoons vanilla extract

2 drops liquid stevia (optional)

1. Place all ingredients in a blender and blend until smooth.
2. Pour into dessert dishes, cover tightly, and refrigerate for several hours.
3. Serve chilled.

⌒ Makes 8 servings

NUTRITIONAL INFORMATION PER SERVING

Calories 108	Carbohydrate 16g
Fat 5g	Fiber 1g
Cholesterol 0mg	Protein 3g

Baked Pears

....

5 organic green pears

1½ cups water

½ teaspoon guar gum

2 tablespoons raisins, chopped

10 almonds, chopped

1 teaspoon cinnamon

2 teaspoons vanilla extract

2 drops liquid stevia (optional)

1. Preheat the oven to 350°F.
2. Wash the pears and slice ½ inch off the top. Set the tops aside. Core the pears with an apple corer without puncturing the bottoms. Place in a baking dish.
3. Place the water, guar gum, raisins, almonds, cinnamon, vanilla, and stevia in a saucepan and heat over medium heat for 10 minutes. The raisins will swell and sweeten the water.
4. Fill each pear with the raisin sauce and replace the top.
5. Bake on a cookie sheet for 30 to 40 minutes, or until soft.

∾ *Makes 5 servings*

NUTRITIONAL INFORMATION PER SERVING

Calories 150	Carbohydrate 32g
Fat 2g	Fiber 4g
Cholesterol 0mg	Protein 2g

Chocolate Mousse

....

2 12.3-ounce packages silken tofu
1 tablespoon vanilla extract
½ cup chocolate chips

1. Place the tofu and vanilla in a blender and process until smooth and creamy. Use a spatula to scrape the sides so that all the tofu is mixed well.
2. Melt the chips in the microwave and pour into blender as soon as they are melted. They will start to harden up again immediately, so it is important to move quickly.
3. Blend again and pour into serving dishes.
4. Serve immediately or chill.

Makes 6 servings

NUTRITIONAL INFORMATION PER SERVING

Calories 100	Carbohydrate 7g
Fat 5g	Fiber 0g
Cholesterol 0mg	Protein 7g

Banana-Blueberry Cream Pie

PIECRUST

3 tablespoons whole flaxseeds

1 cup rolled oats

1 tablespoon hazelnut oil

1 teaspoon ground cinnamon

½ teaspoon ground nutmeg

¼ – ½ cup water

FILLING

1 cup blueberries, fresh or frozen

1 cup low-fat cream cheese

1 tablespoon fresh lemon juice

1 tablespoon vanilla extract

4 ounces silken tofu

1 tablespoon barley malt syrup or honey

4 drops stevia

1 banana sliced

Directions for Piecrust

1. Preheat the oven to 350°F.
2. Place the flaxseeds in a blender and grind to a fine powder.
3. Slowly add oats and mix well.
4. Pour the flaxseed-oat mixture into a bowl and add the remaining ingredients. Mix together.

5. Pat into a 9½-inch pie pan (do not grease), making the crust as thin as possible. Wet fingers periodically so they won't stick to the dough.
6. Bake for 20 minutes.
7. Remove the shell from the oven and let cool.

Filling

1. Combine the blueberries, cream cheese, lemon juice, vanilla, tofu, sweetener, stevia, and half the banana in a blender and blend until smooth.
2. Pour into the pie shell.
3. Slice the remaining half banana and place over the top of the pie.
4. Serve immediately or chill before serving.

Makes 8 servings

NUTRITIONAL INFORMATION PER SERVING

Calories 130	Carbohydrate 15g
Fat 5g	Fiber 2g
Cholesterol 2mg	Protein 7g

Power Cookies

....

1 cup soy flour

1½ cups barley flakes or oat flakes

½ teaspoon baking soda

½ teaspoon salt

½ teaspoon cream of tartar

2 teaspoons ground cinnamon

¼ cup organic canola oil

¼ cup barley malt syrup

1 tablespoon frozen orange juice concentrate

1 egg white

1 teaspoon coconut extract

2 teaspoons vanilla extract

2 drops stevia liquid extract

4 prunes, pureed

1. Preheat the oven to 350°F.
2. Place the flour, barley (or oats), baking soda, salt, cream of tartar, and cinnamon in a large bowl and mix together thoroughly.

3. Place remaining ingredients in another large bowl and mix thoroughly.
4. Add the dry ingredients to the wet ones and mix well. Drop 2-tablespoon balls onto a nonstick cooking sheet and bake for 10 minutes.

~ Makes 20 servings

Note: Stevia is the ideal sweetener for people with diabetes or hypo-glycemia because it is calorie free and does not raise blood-sugar lev-els. Stevia does not break down when heated, so it can be used in baked and cooked recipes.

NUTRITIONAL INFORMATION PER SERVING

Calories 80	Carbohydrate 8g
Fat 3.5g	Fiber 1g
Cholesterol 0mg	Protein 2g

Vanilla Pudding

....

1 12.3-ounce package silken smooth tofu
3 tablespoons water
1 tablespoon unrefined cane sugar
2 drops stevia liquid extract
3 teaspoons maple syrup
2 teaspoons vanilla extract
½ teaspoon guar gum
Pinch of salt
1 teaspoon orange juice concentrate (optional)

1. Place all ingredients in a blender and process until creamy.
2. Spoon the pudding into dessert glasses or bowls.
3. Serve warm or chill in the refrigerator.

~ *Makes 4 servings*

Note: Before measuring sticky liquids such as maple syrup, barley malt syrup, or honey, oil the measuring spoon first. The liquids will then slip out of the spoon easily.

NUTRITIONAL INFORMATION PER SERVING

Calories 83	Carbohydrate 10g
Fat 2g	Fiber 0g
Cholesterol 0mg	Protein 5g

Fruit Gel

3 to 4 tablespoons agar flakes

1 quart apple juice

½ cup raisins

2 cups fresh blackberries, chopped or pureed

1 teaspoon vanilla or almond extract *or* squeeze of lemon

1. Soften the agar in the juice in a saucepan. Add the raisins. Bring the mixture to a boil and simmer for 5 minutes. Stir in the blackberries and flavoring.
2. Pour into a mold and allow to set in refrigerator.
3. Serve chilled.

Makes 8 servings

NUTRITIONAL INFORMATION PER SERVING

Calories 140	Carbohydrate 32g
Fat 0g	Fiber 3g
Cholesterol 0mg	Protein 1g

Blueberry Sauce

....

1 cup blueberries, fresh or frozen
½ cup apple juice
2 teaspoons fresh lemon juice
2 drops stevia liquid extract
1 tablespoon honey
1 tablespoon arrowroot powder

1. Place the berries in a small saucepan with half the apple juice, the lemon juice, stevia, and honey and heat until softened.
2. Remove from heat and process the berries in a blender until smooth. Return to the saucepan and heat over medium-low heat.
3. Dissolve the arrowroot powder in the remaining half of the apple juice, then add to the saucepan. Continue cooking over low heat, stirring, until the sauce is thick and shiny. Remove from heat.
4. Serve hot or store in an airtight container in the refrigerator for up to 1 week. Serve over pancakes or waffles, desserts, or fruit.

Makes 20 servings

NUTRITIONAL INFORMATION PER SERVING

Calories 15	Carbohydrate 3g
Fat 0g	Fiber 0g
Cholesterol 0mg	Protein 0g

Whipped Cream

½ cup whole milk

1 teaspoon vanilla extract

2 drops of liquid stevia (optional)

1. Pour the milk and vanilla in a tall plastic cup and place in the freezer for about one hour. (Cold milk whips more easily.)
2. Remove milk mixture from the freezer and whip with an upright hand blender until peaks form.
3. Add liquid stevia to taste.
4. Chill or serve immediately.

Makes 8 servings

NUTRITIONAL INFORMATION PER SERVING

Calories 10	Carbohydrate 1g
Fat 0.5g	Fiber 0g
Cholesterol 0mg	Protein 1g

Tofu Whipped Cream

....

1 12.3-ounce package silken tofu, chilled
1 tablespoon vanilla extract
3 drops stevia liquid
1 tablespoon honey

1. Place all ingredients in a bowl and blend with an upright hand mixer until smooth.
2. Serve over fruit or desserts.

Makes 15 servings

NUTRITIONAL INFORMATION PER SERVING

Calories 15	Carbohydrate 1g
Fat 0g	Fiber 0g
Cholesterol 0mg	Protein 2g

Glossary

Agar (Agar-Agar): Agar is made from seaweed that is dried and powdered and sold as a thickening or gelling agent. It is tasteless and comes in the form of blocks, powder, and strands. It is widely available in Asian markets, health-food stores, and through mail order sources. It is a good dietary source of calcium and iron.

Apples: Apples are rich in soluble fiber such as pectin. Pectin absorbs water, lowers fat absorption, has cholesterol-lowering effects, and contains antibacterial agents along with antioxidants and anticarcinogens. Pectin is highly recommended for constipation and blood-sugar regulation. Pectins also promote the growth and maintenance of beneficial intestinal flora, which is necessary for proper digestion of food and elimination.

Apricots: Apricots are rich in alpha, beta, gamma, and delta carotenoids, which are all antioxidants. They protect DNA from free radical–induced damage. Dried apricots are exceptionally high in fiber (24 grams of dietary fiber per 100 grams of apricot).

Arame: This brown algae is dark yellow-brown while it is still growing in the sea, black when it is dried. Its blades are about a foot long and wrinkly. It is used fresh or dried for soups and sauces. It is rich in protein, vitamin A, vitamins B_1

and B$_2$, sodium, potassium, iodine, chloride, calcium, and trace minerals.

Bananas: Fiber, potassium, water, complex carbohydrates, and flavor are the banana's key virtues. They are also rich in electrolytes, potassium, calcium, and magnesium. Bananas provide electrolyte replacement and a sweet flavor to desserts. Bananas have a 76 percent water content, which makes them the perfect freezer fruit. Peel a banana and freeze for at least 24 hours. Add 1 frozen banana to a smoothie for a creamy milkshake-textured drink.

Barley Malt Syrup: Sprouted barley liquid is dark brown in color, thick, and sticky like molasses and has a rich malt flavor. Buy only the 100 percent barley products. Many inferior products contain corn malt syrup, which dilutes the flavor and adds more simple sugars. Buy only organic products. Store in a refrigerator and heat the jar under hot water to liquefy when ready to use.

Bioflavonoids: Bioflavonoids are water-soluble compounds, such as hesperidin, rutin, flavones, flavonols, catechin, and quercetin. The main sources of bioflavonoids are lemons, grapefruits, oranges, limes, rose hips, apricots, cherries, grapes, black currents, plums, blackberries, papayas, onions, parsley, legumes, green tea, and red wine. Bioflavonoids help us absorb our vitamin C and assist in the maintenance of collagen, which is an integral part of cells, tissue, and cartilage. Bioflavonoids' main function is to increase the strength of the capillaries, help prevent bruising, hemorrhoids, and varicose veins, and protect against viral and bacterial infection.

Blueberries: Blueberries contain vitamin C, potassium, and natural phytochemicals that prevent infections (bladder), heart disease, and stroke. They also have a lower glycemic index (see definition on page 121) than most fruits.

Brown Rice Syrup: Brown rice syrup is less refined than table sugar and contains many of the nutrients contained in brown rice. Brown rice syrup has an amber color and mild butterscotch flavor. It is not as sweet as white sugar and can be mixed with other sweeteners. Organic products are available.

Carob: Carob is naturally sweet and contains protein, calcium, phosphorous, and some B vitamins. This natural flavoring is similar in flavor to chocolate but does not contain caffeine. Because it's naturally sweet, it does not need sugar added like chocolate does.

Cayenne: Hot red chili pepper flakes (cayenne pepper) are a rich source of B vitamins, PABA, and vitamin C. The cayenne pepper's active oil is called capsicum. It is an energy and metabolism stimulant. It has been used medicinally to improve circulation and treat arthritis, ulcers and sore throats, and digestive disorders involving gas, nausea, or indigestion. It stimulates gastric secretions and peristaltic activity and soothes mucous linings.

Cherries: High in vitamin C, minerals, and phosphorus, cherries have a powerful antioxidant effect and are low on the glycemic index.

Coconut: Shredded or grated coconut and coconut milk are available in reduced-fat or low-fat versions. They are rich in the healthful omega-6 fatty acids. Coconut extract can be used to add sweet flavor to recipes without adding a lot of sugar.

Date Sugar: This sugar is not as refined as cane sugar and contains many of its original vitamins and minerals. Ground dehydrated dates have a coarse, granular texture and a mahogany color. Whole date puree is preferable to the dried sugar product because the puree contains the fiber that reduces its glycemic index. Purchase whole pitted dates and puree them in a blender with water to make a sweetener that can be added to cookies and other baked goods. Dates contain a considerable amount of soluble and insoluble fiber. Always purchase unsulphured, organically grown dates.

Dulse: Dulse is a red seaweed with a pungent, briny flavor. It grows around the British Isles and has a rubbery texture even when dried. Some Irish use it like chewing tobacco. It is primarily used as flavoring in soups and as a condiment on salads and grains. It is available dried, granulated, powdered, or in sheets. It is rich in minerals, magnesium, fiber, vitamin C, beta-carotene, potassium, calcium, iron, and iodine. It is also high in trace minerals and is used as a treatment for thyroid disorders.

Essential Fatty Acids: Essential fatty acids (EFAS) are necessary for brain activity, immune system function, proper skin development, glandular function, and for all of the body's vital organs. They protect the cells from bacteria and viruses. They are precursors to hormone production. They are essential, and Americans generally do not get enough of these healthful fats. There are EFAS in soy foods, nuts, seeds, and flaxseed oil.

Flaxseed: Flaxseed contains lignans, nutraceuticals that inhibit tumor progression and become estrogenic or anti-estrogenic as needed by the body. Raw flaxseed powder, flaxseed oil, and whole flaxseeds are all widely available. Flax adds fiber and essential fatty acids to recipes. Flaxseeds contain both soluble and insoluble fiber. Be sure to drink plenty of water when taking any form of fiber.

All flaxseed products should have a fresh, nutty flavor. If the product starts to smell rancid or fishy, throw it out. Refrigerate all flaxseed products, as they are rich in natural oils that will go rancid if not protected. Flaxseed powder can also be used as an egg replacer. One tablespoon flax powder and 3 tablespoons water equals 1 egg; mix and let stand for 30 seconds.

Ginger: Gingerroot is useful in treating nausea, morning sickness, and motion sickness. Gingerroot also has been used as a digestive and circulatory stimulant for thousands of years.

Glycemic Index: The glycemic index was devised to explain the apparent differences in the blood glucose response to similar amounts of carbohydrate. The standard for the glycemic index is a slice of white bread, which is assigned a value of 100. Each food has its own effects on blood sugar; some raise blood sugar more than others. For example, sweet potatoes have an index of 40 to 49 percent while instant mashed potatoes have a more rapid response with a value of 80 to 90 percent. Soybeans are very low with a value of 10 to 19 percent, which makes them ideal for blood sugar regulation.

Green Tea: Green tea contains numerous health-benefiting phytochemicals and is available in a caffeine-free form as an extract and as leaf tea. Catechins, found in both green tea and black tea, are linked to reduced rates of gastrointestinal cancers. This tea is low in calories and is a good coffee replacement.

Hijiki: Hijiki, a dried black seaweed, has a slight anise flavor and nutty aroma. Usually dried into thin strips, it is available in both dried and fresh varieties at Asian markets, health-food stores, and mail-order companies. All sea vegetables have beneficial fiber, which helps balance blood-sugar levels. Hijiki has a high mineral content and 10 times more calcium by volume than milk, cheese, or other dairy products. It is also high in iron, protein, beta-carotene, B1, and B2.

Holy Basil: The culinary herb holy basil is not the same plant as garden-variety basil. It has been shown to significantly lower blood glucose levels in non-insulin-dependent diabetics without causing side effects.

Honey: Honey contains fructose and glucose, enzymes, and nominal amounts of vitamins and some trace minerals. Honey is less processed than white sugar, which is made from cane and processed with chemicals to clean and bleach it. Collected from flower nectar by bees, it is actually sweeter than white sugar. There are a few drawbacks to using honey as a sweetener. Children under the age of 2 should never eat honey, as it can transmit just enough botulism to be very dangerous to children. Honey also can adversely effect blood-sugar levels, so it must be used sparingly.

Irish Moss (Carrageenen): Irish moss fronds grow along the coast of Ireland and along North America's Atlantic coast. Its stubby, broad, forked fans grow in colors from reddish-purple to reddish-green. Carrageenen is extracted and used as a food supplement and as a thickening agent because it contains calcium chloride. When used as a thickener, the results are a softer and creamier texture than that of agar, but it can be used in place of agar in any recipe. Irish moss is high in iron, beta-carotene, and iodine.

Kelp: Kelp contains easily assimilated iron, potassium, calcium, iodine, and other trace minerals and vitamins. This is particularly beneficial for those with mineral deficiencies that have developed from a long-term fast food diet. It can be purchased dried, granulated, or powdered.

Kombu: The *Laminaria* family of sea vegetables includes kombu. Kombu grows in long, dark-brown to grayish-black fronds up to 15 feet in length. It is harvested and sun-dried and folded into sheets. It makes a flavorful broth. It can be purchased dried in packages and stored indefinitely unopened. After opening, store in a cool dry place for up to 6 months. Kombu is a rich source of beta-carotene, B_2, vitamin C, calcium, and iodine.

Lemons: Lemons contain bioflavonoids, vitamin C, and potassium. These antioxidants are natural anticarcinogens, which help prevent infections, cancer, heart disease, stroke, and high blood pressure.

Licorice: Licorice extract contains many natural chemicals such as coumarins, asparagine, biotin, choline, glycyrrhizin, inositol, lecithin, manganese, paba, pantothenic acid, pentacyclic terpenes, phosphorus, and B vitamins, which give it powerful effects in treating inflammatory diseases, infections, and estrogen imbalances. Glycyrrhizin is 50 times sweeter than sugar, so a little bit goes a long way. Liquid licorice extract and powder are used as sweeteners and tea. They are widely available in the United States.

Maple Syrup: Real pure maple syrup comes from the sap of maple trees and is rich in potassium and calcium. Pure maple syrup has a dark brown color and rich maple flavor. Avoid maple syrups made with added sugar or synthetic sweeteners. Buy only pure U.S. organic syrup.

Miso: *See* Soy for the health benefits of miso, including digestive enzymes and anticancer phytochemicals. Many flavors and varieties are available.

Nori: Nori runs from red to a dusty jade color as it grows. It is 48 percent protein by dry weight and a rich source of vitamins, calcium, iron, and trace minerals. It is the most easily digestible form of seaweed. Paper-thin sheets are made from the seaweed, which can range in color from dark green to dark purple to black. They have a sweet, subtle ocean flavor.

Nori is generally used for wrapping sushi and making rice balls in Japan. It can be purchased toasted (labeled yakinori). It is a rich source of fiber and bioavailable nutrients such as beta-carotene, thiamine (vitamin B_1), and niacin (vitamin B_3).

Nutritional Yeast: Nutritional yeast is a rich source of amino acids, chromium, potassium, phosphorus, magnesium, sodium, copper, iron, zinc, and B vitamins.

Pears: Pears contain potassium, pectins, hemicellulose, vitamin C, folic acid, potassium, manganese, and selenium. Hemicellulose is an indigestible complex carbohydrate or fiber source, which promotes the beneficial intestinal flora necessary for digestion and elimination.

Pectin: High in soluble fiber, pectin is generally extracted from apples but is also found in carrots, beets, bananas, and citrus fruits. It is used as a thickener and binding agent in food products. Pectin can also be used as an antidiarrheal. Pectin is a soluble fiber, which is beneficial in blood-sugar regulation, removing metals and toxins in the digestive tract, and reducing elevated cholesterol and triglyceride levels.

Pumpkin: Pumpkin is high in beta-carotene and has been purported to have benefit for prostate disorders, stomach problems, worms, and morning sickness.

Raspberries: Raspberries are low on the glycemic index (see definition on page 121). They contain natural phytochemicals that help prevent infections, heart disease, and stroke. They also contain vitamin C, calcium, magnesium, and iron.

Sea Salt: Rich unprocessed sea salt contains magnesium, manganese, boron, copper, silicon, iron, sodium chloride, and nickel.

Sea Vegetables: Sea vegetables contain alginate fiber, which reduces the gastric emptying rate in humans with diabetes, aiding in water absorption and blood-sugar regulation. Sea vegetables also contain iodine (necessary for proper thyroid function), omega-3 fatty acids, and fiber. They are a rich source of calcium, iron, magnesium, carotenoids, vitamin C, vitamin E, B vitamins (including B_{12}), amino acids, bromine, and phosphorus. Sea vegetables are available through natural food markets and through mail order.

Soy: Soy foods include soy milk, tofu, miso, tempeh, textured vegetable protein, edamame, and soy protein powders. Soy foods contain calcium, essential fatty acids, protein, and iron. They are a rich source of soluble and insoluble fiber and are cholesterol free and low in sodium and fat. They also contain many substances of medicinal value including diosgenin, beta sitosterol, gamma sitosterol, stigmasterol, daidzein and genistein, phytoestrogens, saponins, phytoesterols, and trypsin. All soy foods contain the phytochemicals known as protease inhibitors, which prevent activation of the specific genes that cause cancer. Protease inhibitors are also known to protect against radiation and free-radical damage.

Soy Milk: With soy milk it is possible to avoid the hormones and antibiotics that are now commonly found in dairy milk. Soy milk is a vegan choice for those who would like to avoid lactose, which is the milk sugar that 30 to 50 million Americans have a hard time digesting. Some people choose soy for the blood-sugar-regulating effects of its fiber or the menopausal-regulating effects of the phytochemicals. Soy milks are available in cocoa, carob, vanilla, cinnamon, and almond flavors, some sweetened, some not. Calcium and vitamin D are added in some soy milks. Soy milk has a higher protein content than rice milk and is available in nonfat, low-fat, and whole varieties.

Stevia: This South American plant extract is an herb rather than a carbohydrate. It is so sweet that a tiny amount is all that is necessary. It is one of the few sweeteners available that does not appear to raise blood-sugar levels. It contains no calories and is an ideal sweetener for people with diabetes or hypoglycemia. It is available in liquid or powdered form.

Strawberries: Strawberries are a rich source of vitamin C and contain potassium, manganese, and biotin. They are also a good source of phytochemicals such as phytoesterols and polyphenols (compounds that may have antiviral activity), and glutathione, a powerful antioxidant and anticarcinogen.

Turbinado Sugar: Turbinado sugar is cane sugar that has not been bleached and highly processed. It contains much of its original vitamins and minerals and does not contain processing chemicals.

Vanilla Extract: Also known as vanillan and ethyl vanillan, vanilla can be used in small quantities adding no fat and just a nominal amount of sugar to a recipe. Use alcohol-free natural vanilla extract for flavoring. Mexican extract is strong and requires just a drop to flavor an entire blender full.

Wakame: Wakame (a kelp) grows in winglike, olive-colored fronds up to 20 inches long in shallow water and up to 20 feet long in deeper waters. The dark brown variety is more strongly flavored. Wakame is high in calcium, iron, beta-carotene, niacin, and protein. It is available through Asian markets, health-food stores, and mail order.

Yogurt: Yogurt is naturally rich in the healthful bacteria needed in our intestines for proper digestion and absorption of nutrients. It is also high in calcium and magnesium. Those who cannot digest other dairy products generally can tolerate yogurt. Plain yogurt is best as it can be purchased free of sugar and additives.

Suggested Reading Materials

Golan, Ralph. *Optimal Wellness* (New York: Ballantine Books, 1995). This book can help you understand the intricate connection among blood-sugar imbalances, food allergies, adrenal exhaustion, nutritional deficiencies, liver toxicity, and poor digestion.

Keane, Maureen, and Daniella Chace. *Bread Machine Baking for Better Health* (Rocklin Prima Publishing, 1994). This cookbook contains recipes for soy bread, spelt bread, gluten-free bread, and wheat-free bread.

Keane, Maureen, and Daniella Chace. *What to Eat if You Have Diabetes: A Guide to Adding Nutritional Therapy to Your Treatment Plan* (Chicago: NTC/Contemporary, 1999). This book is the companion guide to this cookbook. It explains how the ingredients used in the recipes help stabilize blood sugar.

Murray, Michael, Joseph E. Pizzorno, and Joseph N.D. Pizzorno. *Encyclopedia of Natural Medicine, 2nd Ed.* (Rocklin, CA: Prima Publishing, 1998).

Murray, Michael. *Encyclopedia of Nutritional Supplements* (Rocklin, CA: Prima Publishing, 1996).

Resources

Abundant Life SEED Foundation
Box 772
Port Townsend, WA 98368
(360) 385-5660
Sells holy basil seeds, which you can grow in your kitchen.

Body Ecology
1266 West Paces Ferry Road
Suite 505
Atlanta, GA 30327
(800) 478-3842
(404) 266-1366
Sells stevia, kefir, and essential oil supplements

Herbal Advantage, Inc.
Route 3, Box 93
Rogerville, MO 65742-9214
(800) 753-9199
Fax (417) 753-2000
E-mail: smarsden@mail.orion.org
Call the toll-free number for a free catalog or stevia recipe book. Also visit their website at: www.HerbalAdvantage.com.

Kyolic Garlic Supplements
Call (800) 825-7888 for a free sample of Kyolic garlic. Call the garlic hotline, sponsored by Cornell University, with questions about garlic (800) 330-5922.

Multi-Pure Water Purifier

Contact: Tonja Hill (425) 643-2240

Call for information regarding Multi-Pure water purifiers for home use. The purifiers remove lead, chlorine, giardia, and many other harmful substances from drinking water.

The Stevia Company

640 South Perry Lane

Tempe, AZ 85281

(800) 899-9908

Call for a list of stevia products.

Walnut Acres

This farm sells organic produce and products, granolas, soup, and an array of natural products through their catalog. To request a free catalog, call (800) 433-3998.

Cheryl's Herb

836 Hanely Ind. Ct.

St. Louis, MO 63144

(800) 231-5971

Fax (314) 963-4454

E-mail: pawgep@aol.com

This company has a line of stevia products including stevia leaf powder and stevia extract powder.

Roshco Corp.

Call this kitchen appliance company for a free copy of their catalog at (401) 596-5588.

Bastyr University

Nutrition Analysis Services Coordinator

14500 Juanita Drive NE

Bothell, WA 98011

(425) 602-3121
Fax: (425) 823-6222
Have your own recipes analyzed for number of calories; percentage of fats, proteins, and carbohydrates; and micronutrients.

Spectrum Naturals

This company manufacturers high-quality organic oils, vinegars, dressings, condiments, and spreads. Spectrum makes butter replacement spreads that are dairy free, trans-fat free, and primarily organic from soy, canola, flax, and olive oil. They also have a selection of low-fat and low-calorie salad dressings that are appropriate for the diabetic diet. This is one of the few companies that is careful to avoid genetically altered ingredients. Look for Spectrum products in natural-food markets or call to find out where they are sold in your area (800) 995-2705.

SnoPac

This is one of the few companies growing organic green soybeans used for making edamame. Because many of the soybeans in the United States are genetically altered, it is important to purchase only organic soybeans and soybean products. Call (800) 533-2215.

Zyliss Corp.

This company makes my beloved garlic press called the Susi, the most efficient garlic press I have ever used. They also make many other kitchen tools including a can opener that is actually easy to use even for arthritic hands, a handheld spice grinder, and a beautiful citrus peeler. Call (888) 794-7623.

Index